She
Energy

She

Energy

A self-awareness
guide to your
natural energy cycle

JESSICA TERLICK

the kind press

Cover design: Miladinka Milic
Editing: Tegan Lyon
Internal design: Nicola Matthews, Nikki Jane Design

Cataloguing-in-Publication entry is available from the National Library Australia.

NATIONAL
LIBRARY
OF AUSTRALIA

ISBN: 978-0-6455237-2-0
ISBN: 978-0-6455237-3-7 e-Book

My Mum and Dad.
Thank you for always loving and supporting me. You have given me a loving home, lots of opportunities and reminders that I can do it! I love you both so much.

Ben, Ava and Rob.
Thank you for always being my biggest supporters and for loving me for being me. I love you all so much and am so lucky to have our beautiful family.

Indigenous and Traditional Owners

I wish to acknowledge the Traditional Custodians of the land on which I have written this book, the Whadjuk people. I would like to pay respect to the Elders of the Noongar nation, past, present and future, who have walked and cared for the land. I acknowledge and respect their continuing culture and the contributions made to the life and the land in which I now live.

I would also like to acknowledge the six Indigenous seasons Birak, Bunuru, Djeran, Makuru, Djilba and Kambarang.

A note from the author

Regarding gender identity, I wish to acknowledge non-binary and transgender people, and convey that my use of the word 'she' is not intended to offend anyone. My usage of 'she' refers to feminine energy in which all humans have.

On my use of the word seasons, I understand that those who live closer to the equator do not experience the four seasons as I do. Please note that the seasons are used as a way to communicate and identify the 4 stages of your energy cycle.

Contents

Part 1
Align

Part 2
Know your cycle

PART 3
Utilise and flow

Part 4

Share your shine

Introduction

For so long I have questioned who I am, and why I deserve to be happy and have a good life. I have had a burning desire to do more and be more, and yet, I doubt that I am special, worthy or have the ability to be successful. There is also a tiny voice in my head that knows my full potential and yet another voice warning me not to show my true self because it is scared of what people will think. The truth is, no one is thinking of me as much as I think about myself. Those who do think of me would only do so because they love me not because they are thinking I should achieve more in my life. Take this book for example. I have always wanted to write a book. I have dreamed of my book alongside other beautiful authors who felt the need to share what is inside them in the hope that it would help others. I visualise walking into a bookstore in the shopping centre or at the airport and see my book on the shelf. More than seeing it, I feel it. I want it.

I often wonder where my thought patterns come from, especially those focused on success. You may be already aware that our thinking patterns, self-talk, values and emotional responses are developed early on before our hormones kick in. Just as we come to terms with our individuality and understanding our place in the world, we are hit with a huge hormone bomb and left to work through the whole process on our own. I couldn't remember if anyone tried to assist me through my teenage years and even checked with my mum. She simply asked me, 'Would you have listened anyway?' The truth is, probably not, because I felt like I knew what I was doing. In fact, I had mapped out most of my life up until having children. I don't know where this map came from and can only assume it was part of my own perception of what to do with the information I received pre-hormone stage. Essentially, this meant finishing school, going to university, establishing a good career, marrying the perfect guy, having two children, and dividing my time between being a mum and a career woman. So cliché. I wish I had someone there coaching me to look at different options and opportunities, to think outside of what I was conditioned to think was best for me. But even as I write this, I think... would I have listened anyway?

That is why I wanted to write this book. I want to share a range of stories, experiences and strategies to coach you through understanding what happened during the hormone stage that launched you into autopilot mode. I want to create a space for you to think about what you truly want at this point in time and distinguish between your wants and needs and other people's expectations. I want to support you to remove the expectations that you put on yourself and the natural instinct to compare yourself to others. I invite you to use this book as your very own personal development journey. While we learn a lot about subject content at school and strategies for learning, we are not encouraged to learn about ourselves and understand how we operate. Once we dive into how we operate, I want to provide you with the opportunity to investigate what it means to be a woman and how to navigate the monthly rollercoaster of energy and emotions.

The entire world functions on seasons and we have an internal seasonal clock inside of us. Our relationships can even be seasonal as well as our emotions and our learning experiences. By applying this method to our lives, you can then begin to learn how you operate differently to everyone else. This is where I want to enlighten and empower you by teaching you how to use this knowledge to maximise your strengths, address your weaknesses and, most of all, understand when to attempt different activities and tasks and when to avoid certain situations. This is the part where I discuss the true essence of *She Energy*.

Now, I understand that some people may be uncomfortable talking about their period. It took me 15 years to actually understand and appreciate my menstrual cycle and now I use it as my superpower. I also like to talk about it openly with others because I truly believe if we have free communication lines between all women (and men), then having your period will no longer be 'secret women business'.

The journals, affirmation cards and vision board cards that you can also access are tools that will support you along this journey. You are also invited to join our community by following me @jessicaterlick and joining our *She Energy* community via www.jessicaterlick.com.au where you can also access the free materials to support you along the way.

But for now, I invite you to have an open mind and an open heart. Now, what exactly does that mean? As a teacher, I know you will either be someone who loves reading or someone who absolutely hates it and may even take a couple of days to get this far into the book. But hang in there. Keep reading. Keep doing the activities. Keep talking. Keep listening. Allow yourself to learn. You are not being graded on this and there is no way of failing. Although I will talk about minimising competition and comparing yourself to others, there is part of me cheering you on as you read this because if there was a race you would certainly be ahead because you are reading this book. This book is something I wished I had access to when I was younger, and I have hundreds of women in my community who say they wished they had known this 20 years ago! If I knew what I know now, I would have been kinder to myself up until now. Because you know what? We all deserve to live the life we dream of— with great success, achievement and happiness because we are worthy. You are worthy of feeling good and having what you desire!

When I was a young girl, I didn't realise that I had access to *She Energy*. I remember when I first felt the light inside of me and when it was taken away, when it started to dim and I switched to autopilot. After teaching hundreds of young girls, I now realise that this is a common situation. Around the age of 8, our self-awareness activates, and with it, so does our comparison to others. Our societal systems have a lot to answer to when it comes to this, however, it can easily be adjusted with what is happening at home. Young girls are repeatedly told that they are cute, beautiful and 'good'. As they get older, they are still all these things, but they don't often hear it from someone else. These feelings and beliefs need to be felt from within, which is difficult because we have shown our little girls for the last 8 years that they will receive it from the outside on a regular basis. Instead, we want to be encouraging them to learn how to feel and believe it themselves. This is where personal power comes into play. As a teacher I have noticed that by the age of 8, most girls find school a little easier, the rules and routines are something they thrive in but soon it becomes something of competition. Competition with themselves and others.

Imagine yourself as a little girl with a small fire lantern lit inside you. With every little bit of success, that light grows stronger. With every bit of criticism, failure or disapproval, it dims. Take a moment to close your eyes and think about a time when you were younger and imagine the lantern inside. Think of the event and notice how bright the light is. If it was perceived as a positive event, the light is likely going to be bright and big. If the event is perceived as negative, the light is more likely to be dimmed. It would be unrealistic to expect the light to always be bright, however, there are skills and strategies available to strike a delicate balance.

We want our young girls to learn this at an earlier age and the best way to teach them is to learn for ourselves and then lead by example. The first step is switching off the autopilot and waking up to what is happening inside of us.

Now let's take a moment to acknowledge that this book is for all those who identify as a woman. Whether you are premenstrual, menstruating, pre-menopausal or menopausal, you have *She Energy*. *She Energy* is the self-awareness of your natural energy cycle. It is recognising that your body is operating with a hormonal system as well as an external natural system—mother nature! It is the energy system that you can identify, track and utilise. It is the energy system that provides the understanding of why one day or week you feel like you 'have everything together' and the next 'the juggling balls are dropping'. Understanding your natural energy cycle reduces guilt, encourages you to be kinder to yourself and makes you more productive! This book is broken down into four sections:

- ALIGN
- KNOW YOUR CYCLE
- UTILISE AND FLOW
- SHARE YOUR SHINE

You may like to read through the book in one sitting or you may like to stop at each section. There is no right or wrong way to read this book. There is no right or wrong way to learn about *She Energy*. There is no right or wrong way to utilise your *She Energy*. If you would like to explore *She Energy* further alongside this book, you can access my *She Energy* membership at www. jessicaterlick.com.au/membership

I now would like to invite you connect with your *She Energy* before we officially begin.

The Invitation

There is a light inside of you.
Take a breath to make it glow.
Take a breath to make it shine.
Take a breath to make it ignite.

In your heart is a little girl.
She needs you to show her love.
She needs you to show her kindness.
She needs you to show her compassion.

In your heart is a young woman.
She needs your love.
She needs your understanding.
She needs your forgiveness.

In your mind there are a million thoughts.
She needs you to observe them.
She needs you to disconnect from them.
She needs you to release them.
Step forward into the present moment.

Allow yourself to be surrounded by warmth.
Allow yourself to be surrounded by possibilities.
Allow yourself to be surrounded by opportunities.

Acknowledge yourself as your full potential.
Embrace who you were.
Embrace your journey so far.
Embrace who you are today.

As you embark on this journey.
You are invited to connect with yourself.
You are invited to learn about yourself.
You are invited to trust yourself.

Welcome to *She Energy*!

Part 1

Align

Chapter 1

Permission to Stop

It is time to switch that autopilot switch off. There is no need to think 'When Y happens then I will be able to do Z'. Get ready to jump off that hamster wheel. Let us be in the present moment together.

One of the first things you can do to access your *She Energy* is to stop. Can you find moments throughout your day to take some deep breaths? Can you find some moments during the day to check in with your mind, body and soul? Can you find some moments during the day to rest?

When I ask these questions at my workshops, I get mixed responses. It is okay to feel like you can or cannot. The aim is to start small. Make small incremental changes over a long period of time. As you read this book, I invite you to allocate some time every day just for you. You may like to have the time in the morning or evening. If possible, wake up 30 minutes earlier than your household, and allocate that time just to yourself. No need to start your day or do any chores. You may like to have 30 minutes in the evening where you can focus on yourself. Once again, it is not 'extra' time to do some jobs. This time is for you to focus on yourself and be inside your own head.

Throughout this book you will gain some inspiration of what you can do during this time, but for now, just allocate and commit to having at least 30 minutes to yourself each day.

It is hard to stop when you are not used to it. Like a lot of things I cover in this book, when you try them for the first time, they will feel uncomfortable. This is because you are stepping outside your comfort zone when you first attempt them. Your natural response to trying something new is to have second thoughts about doing it. You may even find yourself saying that this is not for you, that it doesn't feel right and that it is not going to work anyway. And you know what? It won't work. It won't work the first time, the second or even the tenth time. It won't work until you practise enough times for your mind to realise that it is safe to do and your comfort zone has expanded. Once you feel safe, you will be in the zone to learn; this is where the magic happens. Nothing changes if you don't make changes. Think of trying something new like stretching an elastic band. When you first stretch the band it feels stiff. The more you stretch it, the more the elastic expands and becomes easier to stretch. If you don't warm up the fibres by stretching them repeatedly then you will not be able to stretch it with ease. When you commit to stopping and allow yourself to have time in your head, you may be at first able to last one minute before you decide that you should be doing other things. You may be able to stretch that feeling to 2 minutes the following day and then 3 minutes the next. Eventually the 30 minutes will end, and you will look for opportunities to have more time to yourself.

You may ask, *why do I want to have this time in my own head?* The answer is to address what is going on inside it—to become a witness to how you treat yourself and recognise how the thoughts you have inform the life you create. It is time to be curious again, to study yourself and your thoughts, to be a student again and benefit from clearing your schedule and prioritising yourself. One of the first lessons I cover in Lead and Inspire is to prioritise yourself again. As women, we have been told that it is our duty to look after others. It is also a natural instinct to nurture. With both 'pressures' together and throwing in the expectations that we 'should' do everything else like keep the house in order, have children, work, exercise, have a beauty routine and so on, this becomes an absolute cocktail—and not one we like! Once we take a moment to prioritise and look after ourselves, take moments to be present and mindful and establish what is important to us, then the cocktail is more likely to be something we enjoy.

When you have an opportunity to take a break and stop, your brain becomes familiar with these pauses. It knows that it has time to reset. It's like recharging, then when you make a decision, you have the highest level of clarity. The decision or thought you come up with is of higher quality because you have used your brain to its fullest potential. Ever spoken to someone whilst on your phone? You hear them, you reply and then they walk away and when you put your phone down you ask yourself if you answered correctly, or you might not even remember what they said or asked. Your brain was occupied and was able to answer at that point in time, but the quality of the answer may have been lower and your capacity to file it away in your memory was not possible because of the volume of information you were taking in at the time.

As I mentioned in my introduction, I turned the autopilot switch on from a young age. I created this switch to be safe. This switch allowed me to focus on what I believed at the time to be most important and then focus all my attention on it. Don't get me wrong, I achieved a lot and was highly successful, but my body paid for it, and I also didn't make decisions with the best clarity. The decisions I made were impulsive and driven by the outcomes rather than the possibilities.

As a result of learning this switch at a young age, I am still able to switch it on at any point. When I was a young adult, I believe this was the only way to achieve because the results were always the same. I would set a goal, do everything in my power to work towards it, forget about time, keep reminding myself that it will be okay once I finally achieve it, then set my next goal because it was like the gap of not having something to focus on was too great. I was missing joy. I was missing looking after myself, and you know what that can lead to. Even though I would achieve while I was in autopilot, I later learned that I was limiting myself. When I made the decisions or took action, these choices were only directed at the outcome. Sometimes this would make things feel like they were taking longer, or I would spend time feeling like a victim. I was basically making life harder for myself rather than enjoy it.

Have you ever driven home and wondered how you got there—did you stop at that traffic light? This is a classic example of being on autopilot. Your brain is split between thoughts and the tasks at hand. You may have been thinking about what has happened during the day or what you need to do when you get home, either way your brain is not focused on the task at hand. Stress survives in the past and thrives in the future. It does not exist in the present moment. There is certainly a time where you can unpack what has happened during the day, in fact, I highly recommend it. Most of the time you know what needs to be done. You prioritise and have a routine of some sort, and anything additional that needs doing could be written down on a to-do list waiting for you. This will help you avoid thinking about the things you have to do when you get home. Then part of your 'getting home ritual' can be to look at your to do-list, no need to think about it in the car.

Back in the 90s, a common strategy of productivity was multitasking. How common is the saying 'Men can't multitask, only women can!' And because it was/is one of the things that women are seen to be able to do better than men, many women see it as a badge to wear with pride. Some of my clients feel that multitasking makes them feel powerful because they are getting a lot of things done at once. Other clients think that it is necessary to multitask because if they don't get it done, who is going to do it? Multitasking is very similar to autopilot. Yes, you will experience success. Yes, you will be able to get all your jobs done. But there will be no end. You will be restricting your ability to finish tasks effectively. You are enabling others to treat you as the go-to person to get things done. You are teaching others that your personal boundaries are very flexible. You are more likely to feel overwhelmed, taken for granted and always busy! I get it—I have been there—and if I am honest, there are times where I go back to this setting. My self-awareness now knows where to stop to interrupt this pattern of behaviour. However, it has taken a lot of time to get to this point and I am hoping by reading this book you will be supported to make this shift too.

Multitasking is like having an internet browser with 10 different tabs open at the top. Each tab has a different topic, some are connected to each other, and some are random. Your brain has the capacity to switch between each tab and organise the information. You know what you want to achieve, and you will end up working out a way to work through all the tabs to finish your task. You may feel a little overwhelmed to begin with, but then as you work through you, start feeling successful by getting tasks completed or finding the information you require. How do you feel afterwards? You may feel tired, after all your brain just had to sort through a lot of information. You may feel hungry, one of your default settings may be to reward yourself with food when you experience success, and you did just complete a big task. You may not feel like talking to others, so when your partner or children go to speak to you, you may not be in the mood and snap at them. I almost want to guarantee that you will not feel satisfied, content or happy.

It is time to switch this autopilot off and close the internet tabs! It's time to stop, prioritise yourself again and tune into what is working and what can be improved! This is your permission to stop.

WHAT DOES ALIGNMENT MEAN TO ME?

Alignment is that feeling of pausing my breath whilst still breathing.

Sitting in the sunlight and feeling the warmth in the rays.

Slipping my shoes off so I can place my feet on the cool grass.

Zoning out of my thoughts and listening to the outside noises.

Allowing my concentration from the outside noises to return to my heart space.

Concentrating on the colour of the glow.

Breathing energy and focusing into that space to make the glow brighter.

Asking the question.

Then listening.

Now take a moment to think what alignment means to you.

LET'S TUNE IN

So much of what happens to us on the outside is a mirror to what is happening inside of us. Have you ever woken up and felt like the day was going to be 'bad' and then hurt yourself getting out of bed or broken something at breakfast time? The internal feeling that something will go wrong has transpired externally. This works in a similar way when we decide we want something like a new car, and then all of a sudden, we start to see that new car everywhere. It is like someone heard that you wanted it and then decided to get it for themselves! We can create the life we want to live on the outside by focusing our attention to creating this reality on the inside.

So, what is your reality like on the inside at the moment? Let's tune in! Take a moment to write down everything you are thinking of right at this moment. You can use your journal or a piece of paper. I like to call this 'Brain Dumping'. You want to release every thought that is currently in your brain. There is no need to judge or think about what you are writing down, just simply write it all out. Now write a list of desired emotions that you would like to feel on a daily basis.

Now shall we bring this energy to life? Read the next set of instructions and then give it a go. You may feel silly doing it the first time, but please just have some fun with it! There is also no right or wrong way to do this.

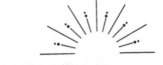

Energising activity

1. Select one desired emotion that you want to feel on a regular basis.
2. Stand up straight, relax your jaw and shoulders and close your eyes.
3. Imagine this emotion has a colour attached to it. It doesn't matter which colour. Just allocate a colour.
4. Now whilst, scanning your body from head to toe, identify where this colour is showing in your body. There might be large areas and there might be small areas.
5. Once you have scanned your body, open your eyes and imagine that colour has turned into a magician's scarf that you can pull from your heart space.
6. Get your hands ready at your heart space and pull (using one hand at a time and alternating) the scarf out of your heart space. Really get your heart pumping by moving your arms.
7. When you feel like you have pulled ALL the scarf out,

scrunch it into a ball. The bigger and emphasised the actions the better.

8. Then stretch it out. Stretch it out to form a large disc.
9. Spin this disc CLOCKWISE. Spin it fast. Spin it faster and faster.
10. Spin it so fast that it takes on a mind of its own. Once you lose control of it…
11. SLAM it back into your heart space.
12. Place your hands on top of your chest and close your eyes.
13. Feel the warmth radiate throughout your body.
14. Breathe into that energy.
15. Imagine that colour taking over your body.
16. Embody that feeling.

You can use this exercise any time you would like to enhance a desired emotion. You may like to do it when you feel negative or have an important meeting or a lot of tasks to do in a day. If you have a heavy feeling that you feel you can't extinguish, you can repeat the same process but spin the disc anticlockwise to change the emotion and imagine a different colour. This changes the energy rather than amplifying it. This is also a great activity to do with your children before school or after they have experienced strong emotions.

So, do you give yourself permission to stop? Can you connect to what alignment means to you and choose to feel that way rather than switching to autopilot? Now that you have a couple of strategies to add to your toolkit, you can have a play around with them during your week to see how you go!

Chapter 2

Journaling

One of the first strategies I teach in the Lead and Inspire community is the power skill of journaling. Many aren't aware of this practice. It still amazes me how many women don't journal. And it amazes me that so many women are surprised that I journal. I wonder if journaling is something we no longer do out of fear that someone will read our diary. When I ask women why they feel like journaling is not something for them, they often respond that they don't know how to, they don't have the time and they are concerned that someone else will read it, because they know that they would have some not-so-nice things to say. I love it when someone says this final point because it is a great segue into explaining why it is so important to journal.

If you imagine those not-so-nice-things as an energy. If you give them a colour, what colour would it be? If you were to close your eyes and scan your whole body as if you were getting an x-ray, where would you see this colour? Crazy how much you can imagine there, isn't it? This is energy occupying your spaces.

Your mental and emotional spaces. You don't consciously know it is there, but it is, and it's draining the energy from you. There are many ways to get this energy out of you, and journaling is one of them. If you just allowed yourself to write it all out—how you were feeling, what has made you feel this way, your ambitions, your dreams and even what you would like to say to others—that energy will be released from you.

I would like you to take a moment to give this a go. You may have a journal or a notebook handy. You may have purchased one of my journals with this book, or perhaps you just have some paper from the printer. Whatever it is, reach for it and write. There is no right or wrong way to write in your journal, just focus on the *why*.

Journaling ⚭ prompts

- What am I thinking about right now?
- How do I feel right now?
- This is what has happened step by step today.
- Things I appreciate today are.
- I am grateful for…

Now let's go back to the activity where I asked you to x-ray your body to scan for that particular colour. What do you notice now? Is there less of the colour? Has the colour changed? See how the simple act of writing down your feelings can change the energy inside of you? Can you imagine how this can impact you when you do it on a flexible-consistent basis? (I will explain what I mean when I say flexible-consistent a bit later on.)

If you would like to start a journaling routine, I recommend writing first thing in the morning. Have you ever woken up in the morning feeling like you haven't slept or perhaps feeling worse off than you did when you went to bed? Your subconscious mind has been processing the information it has been given throughout the day. Sometimes this can bring up events that happened a couple of days ago or even further into the past. By journaling first thing in the morning, you can process all this energy and release it so it you don't carry it into the day. My favourite journal prompts for the morning are:

Journaling 🦋 prompts

- How am I feeling?
- What has caused me to feel this way?
- What am I looking forward to today?
- What is causing me the most *insert feeling*?
- What am I grateful for?
- My focus for the day is?
- How can I be the best version of myself today?
- Is there anything bothering me?
- I remember a time when…
- I would love to…
- I am happy when…
- A boundary I would like to put in place is…
- The solution to this is…

Once this becomes a habit and you are doing it on a flexible-consistent basis (I find that I don't feel like journaling in the morning during my Winter Week, I rather lay in bed and listen to a meditation recording or podcast), you can start journaling at night before you go to bed. This is a great practice to get into as it provides you with an opportunity to process all your thoughts and the day's events before you go to sleep. With all that energy processed, imagine the type of sleep you are going to have. My favourite journal prompts for the evening are:

Journaling prompts

- Today I was happy with…
- My lesson for today was…
- Something that happened today was… and I reacted like… next time I would like to react like…
- This is an area I would like to improve by…
- I am grateful for…
- This person really made me *insert feeling/ emotion* today because…
- I remember a time when…
- In the future I would like to…
- Something I did well today was…
- I am looking forward to tomorrow because…

To those who say to me, I don't have time to journal, my response is, you don't have a *priority* to journal just yet. To give it a go all you need is to set your alarm 15 minutes earlier or select a time in the morning when you have 15 minutes spare. For instance, when your baby is having their morning sleep, or you are having your morning coffee etc. The journaling just has to happen before noon for you to start making it part of your routine.

To those who say to me that they don't want anyone to read

it, I tell them that it doesn't need to be neat, no one needs to read it and you don't need to read it again. You can even choose to have a journal where you can tear the pages out and put them in the recycling. That in itself is so therapeutic.

TIME TO DREAM

When did our goals become too difficult to achieve? Answer: When we continued to move the goal posts. I know you have heard it all before: focus on the journey rather than the destination. I don't know about you, but my inner control freak absolutely detests this saying! It might be the princess in me where I want it now, and I certainly know that the virtue of patience is something I aspire to find naturally. But there is also part of me that simply says, *well why not me?* I want this for you too!

When I first started coaching, I attracted clients who wanted to work on their work/life balance. I soon realised that everyone's perception of a good work/life balance was completely different. I then took this to my live workshops and asked participants to show me how they saw their own work/life balance by making scales with their hands. If your left hand represented your life and your right hand represented your work, and you were playing some form of 'I'm a little teapot' and make scales with your hands, what would the 'balance' look like? Now move your hands to represent how you want it to look. Do you notice and feel the difference? You may like to write your thoughts down in your journal.

Journaling 🦋 prompts

- Where do you feel like you are lacking in life or work?
- What is thriving in work and life?
- What would you like to change?
- What would you like to do more of?
- What would you like to do less of?
- What actually makes you happy?
- Are you living the life you want to live? Why/why not?
- What can you do to align your current reality to your desired life?

The Sun of Life

Let's now dive deeper into looking at each of the separate areas in your life. You may have done something like this before, where it is called the Wheel of Life. I like to shake things up and I changed this to the Sun of Life. It will make more sense shortly.

Take a moment to write down a score for each area of your life. The scoring system is between 1-10, 1 meaning a lot of work needs to be done and 10 meaning that this particular area is exactly where you want it to be. Please do not put too much pressure on what score you give each section. Instead, take a deep breath and just be curious about your score. What is your gut feeling? What thoughts come up when you give the score? You can make some notes along the side that can help with your reflection after the activity.

THE 10 AREAS ON THIS SUN ARE:

Physical environment

Your physical environment is the physical spaces you occupy. These may be your home, car and workspace. You can think of just one area or average all the areas. Just note which areas make you feel good and those that bring the score down.

Finance

How do you feel about your money? How do you feel about the money you currently have? How do you feel about your knowledge money? What is your financial position like? Are you happy with the amount you can spend, save and invest?

Work/career/business

How do you feel about your work? How do you feel about your contribution, career or impact? How do you feel about the work you have to do? What is your work environment like?

Relationships

What is your relationship like with yourself and others? How do you feel about yourself and what do you say to yourself? What type of people are in your support network? Do you have a support network? What is your relationship like with your friends and family? How do you act with your friends and family? Do you have any relationships that are toxic? Do you attract positive people into your life?

Romance

At what level is your self-love? Do you have romance in your life? What is your romantic relationship like with your partner? If you do not have a partner, what is your romantic relationship like with yourself? What does romance actually mean to you? Do you know what romance means to you?

Spirituality

What connection do you have to a higher purpose or power? Do you have time to connect to something outside of your realm? Do you believe in a religion or spiritual practice?

Personal growth/development/learning/education

How much time do you have to learn? how much time and resources do you put into personal development? how do you feel about education? Do you feel like education is important even after you leave school?

Health and wellness

What is your health regime like? How well do you look after yourself? Think about exercise, nutrition, nourishment, supplements, drinking water, sleep, relaxation, stress management strategies, mindfulness activities… basically all the things you 'know' you should be doing to look after yourself and the time and resources you put towards them.

Fun and recreation

How much fun are you having? What do you do that is fun? Do you have any hobbies? What do you do for recreation?

Use of technology/social media/screen time

What is your use of technology like? How does social media make you feel? How much time do you spend on social media? What intentions do you have when you are on social media? How much television do you watch? Are you happy with your use of technology?

This is a great activity to refer to over and over again. Whenever you feel like you need a reset in creating the life you want to live or perhaps you want to check in with where you want to set your goals again, you can come back to this activity. You will also notice that you could do this exact activity tomorrow and your scores could change. As we dive deeper into your energy cycle, you may even notice that if you were to do this activity during a different stage in your cycle you might find that you favour some areas more than others. Just be kind to yourself and allow your current feelings to come out.

Now that you have your scores write your top three:

Now your bottom three:

Take a moment to celebrate your top three, no matter what the scores are, these are the top three areas where you feel your best at the moment! One goal of this book is to encourage women to celebrate more, so please take the moment to acknowledge and celebrate your top three!

Now let's look at the bottom three. These scores are not bad. These scores identify that there is an opportunity to improve. An opportunity to grow. An opportunity to change. How exciting!

If you were to take a moment to brainstorm some ideas, what could you include in your life to just make each score increase by one?

Area:	Area:	Area:

Make a commitment to yourself to integrate some of these things into your week.

It is totally normal to find that your scores change and how you once felt about an area now has a higher expectation because you have enjoyed that level for a certain amount of time. For example, when I do this activity, I find that the areas I scored higher in the previous time have now dropped. This makes total sense! As busy women, we can often feel like we are juggling lots of balls. And sometimes when we drop one, another one can fall as well. The same approach can happen with goals. When we are focusing on three main areas, our focus (and time and resources) goes towards these and therefore the focus can be taken away from other areas. It is only human!

As we get into your energy cycle you can then apply different areas to each stage of your cycle so you have different expectations of consistency. When I first started my teaching career, I knew that reading was super important. It was also my job to encourage my students to read, and yet, I wasn't reading myself (enter all excuses: not enough time, I read enough teaching articles, I was too busy etc.). I would start reading a book and then read it consistently for a couple of days and then put it down on my bedside table and look at it for a couple of weeks. I would even write down 'read' on my to-do list, which would in turn add more stress because I would put pressure on myself to read and then not feel like it at the end of the day (I now call this 'wasting my energy').

Fast forward 8 years later and I had established a consistent reading habit. To me, 'consistently' meant reading during my winter cycle. It made so much sense! I was reading just one week out of each month. The books would sit there staring at me for three weeks, but I now know to avoid worrying or adding reading to my to-do list because the time will come again where I will leap towards it. With this knowledge, I now know that if 'Personal Development/Learning' falls into my bottom three, I schedule to work or focus on this goal in my winter week. That way I am supporting my goal (and my wellbeing) by aligning my goal to my energy cycle.

This brings me to the 10/10 scoring system. Would it be possible to get 10/10 in every aspect? NO. Well, it could be possible because we are giving that scoring criteria, however, it would be unlikely. So, what you want to do is to aim for a range— what range of scores would you be happy with? Remember how I was talking about the work/life balance scales? Same thing applies here. You get to decide what scores you are happy with. As a recovering perfectionist, I believe that it is better to get 10 areas ranging between 8-10 than three areas of 10. But once again, this expectation is something you can come up with.

Now why the sun? The sun is the ultimate star in our sky. The sun and stars shine brightly. When all your life areas are well-balanced and at your desired scores, you will shine brightly too! This is a great activity to complete regularly in your journal, especially when you feel life getting harder. Before you get overwhelmed, you can identify one or two areas you would like to improve. You'll then notice a drastic difference to how you are feeling about life. Journaling is a simple strategy that you can add to your toolkit yet so powerful when it comes to creating the life you want to live!

Chapter 3
Self-Care

Let's start by defining self-care. Admittedly this term is being thrown around left, right and centre, but I am a true believer that self-care starts with making time for yourself. Personal development is taking the opportunity to learn about yourself and connect with your own thoughts and feelings. This is the truest form of self-care. It is up to you what you do during this self-care time. Self-care is not just for Sundays—you should be practising self-care multiple times a day.

One of the metaphors I like to refer to is a rainwater tank. I grew up in small country town in Western Australia and most of the houses I lived in had a rainwater tank attached to the house. I never thought about it at the time, but we always had a filtration system on our taps and my parents would often talk about checking the filters when it was raining so all the beautiful water could be captured. I am so used to drinking filtered water that when I away on holidays I have to pack my own bottled water. What a princess! And I love it!

It wasn't until I was reflecting on how I felt early in my teaching career, where I would get home from work and crash on the couch, begging myself to get up and then not moving until I had to get ready for bed. I was exhausted and this was without children or a partner! I had exerted all energy by the end of the day. I operated on school terms, so I would be fine for 6-7 weeks and then fall sick in week 8, push through until school holidays, fall sick again, take a week to recover, use the second week of the holidays to plan and get ready for school and then repeat the cycle again. I wish I knew what I knew now about my energy cycle. I was a rainwater tank; I would fill myself up with very little and then 'pump' what I had left out to those I served: my students. I had nothing left for anyone else and I certainly didn't have anything left for myself.

Here is the thing with rainwater tanks, when the water is gone, only sludge is left at the bottom. When a little water is added, the sludge may mix a little then get pumped out. Now, the filtration system may remove the sludge, but this also takes more effort and energy. And what type of water (service or product) are we really producing if we are pumping from the bottom of our rainwater tanks? So, when I explain self-care to my clients, I talk about it being like a rainwater tank. We want to fill ourselves up with the most beautiful rainwater, so we overflow to others rather than pump 'what we have left'. You may even like to take it one step further and say that we want our rainwater tanks so full that the 'sludge' is slowly removed because of the healing work that we do, which in turn filters out because there is so much water! Self-care for the win!

To introduce more self-care into your life, I like would like to encourage you to create a self-care menu where you can simply write down all the tasks you enjoy doing and then select what you would like or need to do when it comes to your self-care time. During the four different stages of your cycle, you will notice that you feel like doing different self-care activities.

I have included a copy of a self-care menu that Lead and Inspire Community members put together and a blank one for you to create yourself. You may like to visit www.jessicaterlick. com.au/sheenergy to download a digital copy of all the extras included in this book.

Self-Care Menu

Energising Activities	Calming Activities
Do an exercise class	Listen to a guided meditation
Play your favourite song	Go for a walk
Turn the music up and dance or sing loudly	Play with a pet
Listen to a podcast	Play with your children
Make a nutrient-filled smoothie	Call a friend
Catch up with friends	Run a salt bath
Book a date with a loved one	Take a moment to journal

Step outside your comfort zone	Take a moment to read
Go for a bike ride or hike	Cook your favourite meal
Learn something new	Run a foot spa
Teach someone else something new	Go outside and experience nature
Declutter a room or cupboard	Deep breathing *(even download a breathing exercise)*
Do something that makes you laugh	Have a short nap
Have a meaningful conversation with a loved one	Watch a movie or television show *(without looking at your phone or doing something else)*
Take your shoes off and walk outside on the sand or grass	Colour i/paint or be artistic
Book some time off work	Plant a herb garden
Turn off your phone	Stretch your body
Prioritise your to-do list	Drink warm lemon water
Move your body	Have a cup of tea

Use some invigorating essential oils	Make a veggie full soup or slow cook something
Take a cold shower	Watch a campfire or fireplace *(you can even watch a YouTube video clip)*
Take a 15-minute break	Sip wine or drink of choice from your 'special occasion' glassware
Write a list of everything you have completed/achieved today *(Yes, getting out of bed is one, bonus points for making your bed)*	Give yourself a manicure or pedicure
Start a gratitude journal	Moisturise your feet and then put socks on before going to bed
For an extra treat	**For an extra treat**
Buy nourishing vitamins	Book a day spa package
Hire a house cleaner	Book a float tank
Attend a workshop on a topic you love	Attend a yoga class
Visit the hairdresser	Book a massage

The next thing to do is to recognise what self-care means to you and only you. You may see different forms of what self-care can look like on the internet or social media. You may even say you would like to do those things. However, what you will benefit from the most is identifying what will work best for you. Self-care does not always mean beautiful, relaxing baths and getting your nails done all the time. Self-care is also about the care you have for yourself. What personal boundaries can you put in place to look after yourself? What can you say no to more often? What can you say yes to more often?

I named my company Lead and Inspire after I learnt the importance of leading by example. As Ava was growing up and started to take notice of what I was doing, I recognised how much of a 'sponge' her brain was. As the saying goes 'monkey see, monkey do'. This made me think about how I want Ava to treat herself when she is older. And of course, I want her to look after herself. So, I need to teach her that. As women, it is important for us to teach our children that we are important enough to look after ourselves and that there are numerous ways we can look do this.

Now I can hear you, where can you find the time for more self-care? Giving yourself permission to stop is an example of self-care. Selecting one thing off the menu and giving yourself a week or even a month to do that one thing will make a difference. All you have to do is start. When you sit down to plan your week or write in your diary, have a printed copy of your own self-care menu nearby and add a couple of activities to your week.

When I first started focusing on introducing self-care into my life I really struggled. I had a toddler and a home to look after, and I felt like all my time should be spent looking after both. I began to think about how I could bring self-care into my current reality and prioritise it more. It is never that we don't have enough time, we simply don't prioritise self-care.

After journaling and thinking about what I wanted to do, I got myself a packet of sticky notes and numbered them from one to 21. At the time, I'd read that it took 21 days to make a habit. I now know that the amount of time does not matter. What's most important is how you integrate this habit into your day or life. This is what makes it stick. Performing the same task consistently allows you to see what works and what doesn't. If it is something that is worth having, you will eventually work out how to integrate it into your life. The 21 days worked well for me. My habit was to do something that looked after me every day and then write it down on the sticky note before going to bed. It worked brilliantly. I didn't have to follow any structure or routine. I had flexibility in what I could choose and the new habit I was forming was to think about looking after myself during the day.

I cannot remember all the benefits I experienced over the 21 days, but I can remember feeling better about myself and having more time to get things done. I think the most noticeable benefit was that I could think clearly. A lot of my self-care tasks were about sitting quietly with myself or journaling my thoughts, exercising and going for walks—all things that clear my mind.

On the flip side, there was guilt and questions. As I started to do more self-care tasks, I began to feel guilty for spending time on myself. It was like something was programmed in me to say that I was a mum now and my focus needed to be entirely on my child. And then there were questions from my loved ones: *why are you doing that? What do you need that for? What are you trying now?* It wasn't like I was already up against it in my own mind that I started to get questions from others. I truly believe what got me through this stage was surrounding myself with other women venturing on the same journey, one where they decided to look after themselves, not only because they deserved it, but because would benefit everyone around them. Once this stage passed, not only could others see the benefits I was experiencing they could see the benefits in Ava and at home. I exuded a certain level of calmness; I was enjoying life and I liked the way I looked in the mirror.

It may take time to feel like it is totally okay to look after yourself. Just like it will take time to form habits. To simplify this process, set one habit; aim to select one (or any number you like) item off your self-care menu every day. Imagine what a difference that will make!

Chapter 4

Self-Awareness

You are actually in control of your thoughts and what you attract in life! Once you give yourself permission to pause, start journaling and introduce self-care into your life, you will begin to notice that you will generate more self-awareness. Self-awareness is the ability to recognise how you are feeling, what you are thinking and completely detach from yourself. This is essentially looking inward, witnessing yourself experience emotions and then analysing with no bias.

To introduce you to this concept, take a moment to list the emotions you feel on a regular basis and then list the desired feelings you want to feel. You can draw lines across the table to show the feelings you experience on a consistent basis and if they are desirable.

Journaling ⚘ prompts

- How do you feel most of the time?
  (Brainstorm all your feelings and make note of the time, day, and the activity you are doing before, during or after.)
- How do you want to feel all the time?

YOUR DESIRED FEELINGS

All emotions are neutral. They are neither good nor bad. I know I refer to them as positive and negative, but this is because we, as a society, label them like this. However, from this point forward I will refer to them as desirable and less desirable. It is important that we still feel the less desirable emotions to not only experience them but to recognise the contrast experience of a desirable emotion. If we felt desirable emotions all the time, they would soon become less desirable because that would be our new normal. Our brains are always seeking more.

Now that you have taken the time to identify your desirable emotions, can you list the activities that make you feel this way? How often are you feeling this way and how often are you doing these activities? I am sure there will be a direct link. If you were to commit to doing at least one of these activities a week, how would that make you feel?

Let's take a moment to look at your week. During my workshops I like to have participants highlight and break down their week. You may like to start by showing when you go to bed and when you wake up in the morning. You can then allocate the time you spend getting ready in the morning, household chores, parental duties (if you have them) and meal preparation time. If you have different types of work, you may like to break these down specifically and then you can get one step closer to identifying when you have relaxing time. During this relaxing time, are you really relaxing or are you still overloading your brain with information by being in front of the television or on social media? As you do this activity, allow your thoughts to come to the surface and see what light bulb moments you have. Is there any time you are spending on tasks that can be delegated? Or perhaps you are using them as a way to feel busy or procrastinate. How much time do you have allocated for yourself? Do you have any time to wind down or rest? Can you already see how you could time block certain activities according to your cycle or is your week very structured? Do you have space for changes, fun and spontaneity?

	MON	TUE	WED	THU	FRI	SAT	SUN
12am							
12:30am							
1am							
1:30am							
2am							
2:30am							
3am							
3:30am							
4am							
4:30am							
5am							
5:30am							
6am							
6:30am							
7am							
7:30am							
8am							
8:30am							
9am							
9:30am							
10am							
10:30am							
11am							
11:30am							
12pm							
12:30pm							
1pm							

1:30pm							
2pm							
2:30pm							
3pm							
3:30pm							
4pm							
4:30pm							
5pm							
5:30pm							
6pm							
6:30pm							
7pm							
7:30pm							
8pm							
8:30pm							
9pm							
9:30pm							
10pm							
10:30pm							
11pm							
11:30pm							
12am							

Now that you have taken the time to break down what you are currently doing, take a moment to brainstorm what you would like to continue to do, remove and delegate. Once you have reflected on this, you may like to take the time again to do another time blocking chart to see if you can make some changes now.

GET OFF YOUR PHONE
(AND I SAY THIS WITH THE BIGGEST SMILE)

Assess how much you use your phone. How often are you checking it? How often do you feel the need to look at it? What are the first apps you open? One of reasons women come to me for coaching sessions is because they feel like they don't have enough time or energy to be doing what they want to do. When we start to track what they are spending time on, we realise that the amount of time spent on their phone and in front of the television could be used doing the things they would like to do.

In 2017, I trialled not watching television at night. During this time, I wrote in my journal, sat outside, read books and went to bed earlier. Before this, I would sit down to watch television at night and then go to bed. I felt like I did not have enough time to do anything because once dinner was done, the kitchen was tidy and the kids were in bed, it was then my time to watch television. Oh, how wrong I was. It was my time, and it was my time to do what I wanted. Sitting and watching television may be something you want to do, but please don't restrict yourself. Try something different every night. The main thing is, whatever you choose to do, choose it with intention.

In 2018, I found that my business was getting really busy, and I was on my phone a lot. When I did my yearly reflection at the end of December, I realised that I was using up a lot of my time on my phone and missing out on quality time with the kids, never completely listening to what they were saying. I don't care who you are, if you are looking at your phone when someone is talking, you are not listening. So, I decided to put my phone on charge in the office, turn off all notifications and check my phone at specific times. That way, I am fully focused when I am looking at my phone and don't end up going down the social media rabbit hole.

In order to create the life you want to live, you really need to look at what you are doing now and create space for what you want to introduce. Your phone and television usage can really open a lot of space for you.

I now watch television every night with my husband, Ben. This is intentional because he likes to watch television with me, and I see it as a way for us to spend time together. However, I will have nights where I am reading, working in the office, doing some stretches, drawing with Ava or playing with Rob.

NOW LET'S DIVE EVEN FURTHER INTO WHO YOU ARE AND WHAT YOU WANT!

Who do you want to be? What do you want to do? What do you want to have? While these are three classic coaching questions, they are undeniably powerful. If you were to answer these three questions on a daily basis in your reflection journal, your brain would collect enough data to start searching for these things and bring the opportunities to you. So let us take a moment to answer these three questions below. Remember, like all questions, the answers can change at any point in time and just because you write them down, it does not mean they are set in stone.

Who do you want to be?
What do you want to do?
What do you want to have?

We will revisit your brainstorm in the next chapter. For now, take some time to review what you have written. You may like to add things over the next couple of days or week. You may like to ask others around you what they would like to do, who they would like to be and what they would like to have. Please do not share what you have written unless you know that the person will just listen, there is no need to set yourself up for receiving and unnecessary judgement. When I do this activity and start searching outside of myself for suggestions, I often don't share what I want until I am crystal clear myself.

HOW TO OBSERVE YOURSELF

I love people watching. I could sit for hours in a shopping centre and watch people walk by. I think over time I have developed an almost hypervigilance when it comes to 'people-watching'. However, by doing this I have been able to flip it around to prompt myself to look inward. Why was I so curious to watch what others were doing? Even as I write this, I am not entirely sure, however, I do know that I previously judged and compared myself to certain people that would 'trigger' me. When I say 'trigger' it is not always referring to a negative emotion. They might trigger feelings of inspiration. A trigger is simply a sign from your subconscious saying that there is something here that you need to observe and recognise. So, this is a great starting point to observe yourself. When do you get triggered? Who triggers you? What triggers you?

Social media is a real 'comparison highway'! Rather than scrolling through social media and allowing yourself to feel miserable and 'triggered', look at it as a personal development journey. Grab your journal and let's dive deeper!

Journaling 🦋 prompts

- What do you see that triggers you?
- Why do you think you reacted in that way?
- What is it that you need to heal or address?
- What is it that you want?
- Why do you want that?
- Why do you not want that?
- Can you remember a time that this happened when you were younger?
- Is this a pattern that happens regularly?
- How would you like to move forward from this?
- What can you learn from this?
- What actions can you make next?
- Is this anything you want to add to your 'be, do or have'?

The best way to learn about yourself is to give yourself time to observe and reflect. Allow this process to be part of your journaling. Have fun with it. You may find some things need to be unveiled at a deeper level, if this is the case, add different experts, healers, doctors, psychologists, support lines, kinesiologists, coaches and mentors to your self-care menu.

WATCH HOW YOU SPEAK TO YOURSELF

I first started to recognise how I spoke to myself when I started exercising on a daily basis. It was an ongoing battle of *I don't feel like this, I can't do this, I am never going to get better* and *this is just way too hard*. I was adamant that I would achieve my goals, so I just kept saying to myself, be quiet, show up and do the work. This eventually took over the other battle in my head and it became easier to show up and do the work.

At the same time, I was reading *Open Wide* by Melissa Ambrosini and learnt about my 'inner mean girl' (Melissa has a specific book about this if you would like to check it out). As I continued to investigate my inner mean girl, I came across other terms like ego and conscious and logical brain. This is the part of the brain that wants to keep us safe. It is programmed according to every experience we have had: a time where we were laughed at for something when we were younger or hurt after putting ourselves out there. The instinctual reaction is to avoid the experience in the future. This is the part of the brain that shapes our comfort zone. The more comfortable we are, the louder the voice and the less likely we are to change. To overcome this inner mean girl, I first had to be aware of her, know when it was her speaking in my head (the ultimate self-awareness), and then I had to recognise her. It is not that we have to silence her completely, it is just to recognise what she is saying, question if it is true to you and then look for ways to re-program what she is saying. This expands your comfort zone, gives you a new way to react or be proactive, and genuinely makes you feel better about yourself because you are aware of how you are speaking to yourself.

I have a lot of students who come to my classroom at the

start of the year who still do not recognise that they are their own individual separate from their family unit. They have the ability to think and act independently, and these decisions have either negative, positive or neutral consequences. Not all consequences are negative. Do you remember going through school and thinking, *when will I need to know this later in life?* My answer to that is, while you will very rarely need to remember it, what you gain from learning it is the fully functioning and firing neural pathways that you will use when you are older. The sooner that we recognise that learning is not all about the content and rather the skills we gain when we learn effectively, we will feel the full potential of our capabilities.

Our patterns and behaviour are quite often learnt from those we look up to when we are younger—most commonly our mother and father figures. I would like to go a step further and say teachers as well because of all the time we spend with them. If you were to take a moment to write down all the impactful words you remember from these significant figures then predict what they think about themselves, could you see a connection to the patterns and behaviours you have today?

My dad loves to celebrate and commemorate with food, and I absolutely love him for it! Guess what I now like to do? Yes, you've got it. I eat to reward and celebrate, as well as to deal with my emotions. When I became a mum, I noticed that I was passing this behaviour onto my kids and realise it is a lot harder to keep the behaviour for myself and do it differently for my children. The hard work is easier (but still hard) when I change my patterns and behaviour and then this naturally transfers to the children.

One of the most powerful ways to change your patterns and

behaviour is to change your thoughts. I was coaching a girl in netball who would put herself down when she missed a goal. The thing was, she didn't even realise when she was doing it. She would say 'dang it' in a humorous way which resulted in her team members laughing. I pulled this observation to her attention, and she said that it was better than them being upset with her for missing the goal. While this is understandable, I felt something so simple could escalate as she got older. So, I became curious and observed her behaviour and the way she carried herself. She very rarely smiled but would often have those around her smiling with her comments, quite often at the detriment of herself. I asked her one day if she believed what she said about herself. She went to say no and then she paused and said that she did a little bit and then continued to say that yes, it was actually true! I told her this wasn't true but if she kept thinking it and saying it out aloud, she would start to think it. When I asked her if she wanted to feel this way about herself, she said no, and I told her we would start on the netball court. After coaching her for a couple of weeks I started to notice she was smiling more, and her friends were smiling with her, and she was noticeably standing taller. When she missed a goal she cheered and rallied her teammates, knowing that it was just part of the game.

I know that this may be a powerful enough example to show you how your thoughts affect your reality, but this is not the only reason I selected this example. See, I met her mum briefly one day when we were having a friendly practice game. The team didn't perform to their best, but it was a good learning opportunity with lots of teachable moments. When we were walking off court, I noticed the look on the girl's mother's face.

She was very grim. I smiled at her, and she shook her head saying that it was a waste of time for her daughter. Trying not to respond with my first initial emotion (complete irritation and defensiveness), I paused and waited for her daughter to catch up with us. I then asked if she thought it was a waste of time, she didn't believe it was a waste of time at all and listed all the positive things that came of the game. She smiled at me and said that she had fun and was just glad to play a game of netball.

As you can imagine, this stuck with me for the rest of the afternoon, I really wanted to just hand the mother a business card and say *I would love to work with you* because I genuinely felt like I could help. I didn't do this for two reasons: 1) she was not yet ready to work with me because she was caught up in her own world and not even aware how much it was affecting her daughter; and 2) we teach best when we lead by example rather than directly approach, lecture or assume someone needs to learn something.

Self-awareness can start at any time after the age of 8. All you have to do is start to become curious with your thoughts and feelings. Don't be afraid to ask for what you want and watch the way you speak to yourself. When you feel a strong emotion, take the time to step back and examine it. Self-awareness is a skill that takes time to build and develop. Allow yourself to grow. We can all start teaching ourselves and our children how to become more self-aware.

Chapter 5

Positive Affirmations, Visualisations, Vision Boards and Incremental Changes

Why are we always waiting? *I'll just do this and then I can do this. Once this is done then I can have/do that!* Many women automatically serve and put the needs of others before our own (until we started reading this book). How often do you go shopping and easily buy for your children or partner but struggle to find something for yourself? What does your underwear drawer look like? A great way to tell if you are placing a priority on yourself is by looking at your underwear drawer or even your pyjamas. How old are they? Do you need to throw some out? Do you need to buy some new ones? Do you even like them? Are they supporting you? (Funnily, these are almost identical to the list of reflection questions I am going to ask in the 'Positive Relationship' chapter!) You have permission to upgrade your underwear and pyjamas this week. You will no doubt be surprised at the difference it makes!

Time to revisit what you wrote down in the last chapter. Have you had enough time to marinate in all your possibilities? This is the time to be truly honest with yourself. It doesn't matter if there is no perceived way that you can achieve or have what is on your list. There is no one marking you and there is no due date. The only person judging what is on that dream list is you. Notice how those things make you feel. What are you telling yourself about the things on the list? Do you believe you can achieve them or are you saying that it is not possible? What is your inner mean girl saying? Remember there is a lot we can learn about ourselves when we question what we are telling ourselves. Please dream big when you work through this chapter. We are going to lean into making magic happen so you are closer to what you actually want to be, do and have!

VISUALISATIONS AND VISION BOARD

It is now time to really get clear on your ultimate life, that is, the life you want to create. It is the life where you are who you want to be, do what you want to do and have what you want to have. So, take a moment to visualise this. You might like to take some time in your journal to write what it would look like. At the end of each year, I release my *Leap into *insert following year** e-book. You can download it from my website if you would like to use it for this part of the planning.

Once you are clear on your ultimate life, you now want to collect validation and visual things to remind you. I love to create a vision board. Take some time to collect images that represent your ultimate life. You can print these out or digitally create your vision board. Then find a place to put it on display, somewhere you can see it on a daily basis. The idea of a vision board is to visually see what you are working towards. This rewires your brain to look for opportunities, validation and examples of what you see on your vision board in real life. It also supports one of the universal laws: the law of attraction. When you want to attract something into your life, you need to send signals to your brain of what you want to attract. Kind of like the 'cookies' on your phone when you visit websites. You searched for something whilst browsing and then all of a sudden your social media feed is flooded with advertisements relevant to your search history.

The first time I created my vision board I was really nervous to let anyone know. I was worried what others would think of me. Especially my husband. I created my board using images I printed out and put it together on an A3 piece of paper. I was very vulnerable and defensive about what I had put on there. I already had my inner mean girl telling me that it was not possible and reminding me that it was a silly thing to do. I now know that this is because she was trying to keep me safe from disappointment and because we grew up thinking that 'dreams cannot come true'. So, I took a courageous move and asked to buy a small pin up board. Yes, I was a woman in her thirties with two children, working part-time, and I asked permission to buy a product less than $50—absolutely ridiculous— but that was where I was on my journey at that point in time. I was doing my best with the resources I had.

Just when I thought I had made the most courageous decision, I then had to ask if I could put it up on the wall in our walk-in robe. By this stage, I had more issues with putting it up in the house to be seen than my husband did! Once the pin up board was up, I pinned my vision to the board but didn't look at it for a couple of weeks because I was still judging myself. I felt like now I had put it up, if I didn't get everything on that board, I would be a failure. But once I overcame this fear of failure, I started to view it as simply having fun. It was fun to look at the board, it was fun to dream, it was fun to visualise, it was fun to journal about, it was fun to think about it. How fun it was to have a 'hidden' vision board.

At this point in time, the magic started to happen without my realisation. See, as I started looking at the vision board, thinking about the things that were on there and journaling about possibilities, I naturally started creating plans. These plans led to me taking actions and then the actions led to me bringing some things to life on my vision board. This was only the beginning to the magic. When I started noticing that I was achieving or getting what was on the vision board, I started to create more plans and take more action, and then my husband started to notice that my vision board was coming to life.

At the end of the year, I decided to repeat the process I have shared with you in these last 2 chapters. I was so thrilled to have achieved things that were on my board. I kept some of the images to put up on my new board and printed some different ones. I also noticed I did not achieve all images on my board, but I did not want any more. I had trialled to see if it was what I wanted, and at some point it was, but now, it was no longer relevant to my ultimate life. That's the thing, we don't know what we don't want until we try it out. My second vision board required Blu Tack to stick additional A3 pages on the wall! I now have two vision boards: one in my office (on view for everyone to see) and one in my walk-in robe. Sometimes my board lasts a year, sometimes a season. I just know when I need to change it and I allocate time to dream and visualise it again.

POSITIVE AFFIRMATIONS AND ANCHORING

As you would have seen with my vision board journey, I had to re-wire what I was telling myself. I have always been naturally positive and sought for solutions rather than excuses. As a teacher and coach, I naturally gravitate towards being a cheerleader. I now needed to be my biggest cheerleader.

When I was 9 years old, my dad came back from a conference he had been on and gave me a printed copy of a document (now known as an e-book) that was called *You can do it*. My dad had obviously noticed my change in belief in myself. I did not read this document straight away. Instead, I kept it in one of my piles (piles are part of my organising regime—more on this later). I did not read this document until I was 15 after my hormones had settled right down. I remember laughing to myself that I really should have read it when my dad gave it to me because I have learnt what it had said without reading it and it would have fast-tracked what I had to learn by myself if I had just read it. But would it have really? The title 'You can do it' was actually enough and all I needed to believe that I could do it. I just became aware of the process (and what the document outlined) after going through the process myself time and time again. 'I can do it' is an automatic positive affirmation that has fuelled a lot of my achievements over time. So, one of my first positive affirmations that went on my vision board was 'I can do it'.

I also trialled different ways to introduce new positive

affirmations into my sub-conscious brain. When I wanted to make huge changes to my thoughts, I started to write positive affirmations on post-it-notes and carry the note around me with me for the day. Every time I reached into my pocket, I would pull it out and say the affirmation either aloud or in my head. I also have positive affirmation cards that I pull to give me new inspiration of the different ways I can think. I love to do this with my kids as well and I even have a deck for them. When we give our brains something to connect to and a different way of thinking, it looks for the ways to reinforce this thinking and as an effect, we end up feeling or experiencing something that makes us feel this way.

My latest vision board has a variety of positive affirmations all over it and I have made it part of my daily rituals to read them. I love when my inner mean girl brings something to my attention and then I respond back with a positive affirmation. So powerful!

INCREMENTAL CHANGES OVER TIME

Now that we have the vision and the positive affirmations, let's look at the action part. We have to create space for the new! Introducing decluttering. You might have heard about decluttering and Marie Kondo asking if items bring you joy. What I would like to introduce is having a different type of 'why' when decluttering. That 'why' is so we can create space for your ultimate life. Our comfort zones are not only just inside of our heads, but they are also in our physical world. We surround ourselves with what makes us comfortable. This comfort keeps us safe or supresses what we don't want to deal with.

My first experience with decluttering was actually exercise:

I decluttered a lot of mental and emotional baggage, while improving physical strength. The sweat and tears I experienced were the most therapeutic way to declutter! As I gained more energy, I started to go through every room and drawer in the house. My philosophy was, does this fit into my ultimate life or is it a stepping stone towards it? Some things would stay, and other things would be donated or thrown out. I would have a list going of what I needed to buy or upgrade. As I was going through this process, I really felt like I was 'stripping' back. I was becoming aware of what we really needed and what we were spending our money on. Before I bought something, I really questioned if it was to just make me feel better right now or if it was something that was part of my ultimate life or something that would bring me one step closer.

Decluttering not only makes you feel really good, it makes your house easier to clean. Decluttering regularly each gets easier and quicker and easier every time. Going through the process also reminds you of what you have to upgrade and before you know it, you have created a space with things you actually like that have purpose, look good and are high quality. The process also saves you a lot of money and you can even make money if you are able to sell the things you have.

The most significant feeling I experienced when decluttering was the release of energy. I felt spacious. I felt organised. Doing things around the house didn't take me as long so I felt like I had more time. Not worrying about where things were, not using things I had or thinking I wanted something better gave me the feeling of having more energy!

The next step to decluttering is anchoring in your ultimate life. I was introduced this term by one of my mentors, Denise

Duffield-Thomas, who also highly recommends decluttering and upgrading. I joined her Money Bootcamp after reading her book *Get Rich, Lucky Bitch*. In Money Bootcamp, I learnt about anchoring what you want your life to be like. You can do this is a variety of ways:

- Create a screen saver or backdrop to your phone or computer.
- Buy an item that signifies the life you want.
- Visit the display houses you want to build or drive through the neighbourhood you want to live in.
- Get prices for the items you want.

It can be so fun to anchor what you want to create more of in your life. I love seeing all my anchors around my house and workspace as they are timely reminders of the life I am creating.

THE FORMULA FOR MAKING YOUR DREAMS COME TRUE

If I was to tell you that there was a magical formula to make all your dreams come true, would you want to know what it was? I highly recommend you read *Make It Happen* by Jordana Levin because she comprehensively explains how to make the law of attraction work for you!

Here is a version of the formula:
Thoughts + feelings + actions + trust = creation

Thoughts

As you can see, creating your ultimate life begins with your thoughts. What do you think you want to have, do and be? Write down what you want in your journal. Start to talk to people about what you want. Write down your intentions (I use intentions rather than goals).

Feelings

Then you can tap into how you want to feel. What would it feel like to have, do and be everything you desire? What positive affirmations can you refer to that anchor your ultimate life? What are your desired feelings?

Actions

Your actions are not just what you 'have to do'. They are not just the 'action steps' to reaching your goals. I want to avoid framing 'achieving' in such a way. Goal setting is so 90s! Setting intentions with purpose and feeling comes with more feminine energy. See action as a way to flow forward rather than push. What can you do to feel the way you want to feel? What can you do to take one step closer to your intentions? See how much better that feels?

Trust

Patience is not my strength, so it would not be right of me to say you have to be patient. However, I am capable of trust. So, I implore you to trust that you can make it happen, trust that there is a higher purpose, trust that there is magic out there to support you, trust that you do have everything inside of you to make things happen. You are doing the best you can with the resources you have right now. Trust that in your journey you will collect and learn new resources to build on your current repertoire of strategies and then you will have more resources to call upon.

See this formula as a process. You can even trial it on the smallest of things, even materialistic things. Have fun with it. Whenever I want to create something new in my life, my automatic feeling is fun. If I am having fun, then I am creating the life I want to live. List the emotions you feel on a regular basis and then list the desired feelings you want to feel. You can draw lines across the table to show the feelings you experience on a consistent basis and if they are desirable.

What key emotion do you want to think about when you are creating the life you want to live?

Chapter 6
Emotions and Forgiveness

All emotions are normal and necessary. The balance is whether they are helpful or unhelpful. Anger is my default emotion and my body's response is crying when I am experiencing anger in an unhealthy way. The catch with this is, I then become frustrated from crying instead of communicating effectively, which leads to more anger and then, you guessed it, more crying! I am still working on my emotional intelligence, particularly recognising my emotions.

What I have learnt so far is:
1. That emotions are neither good nor bad.
2. Knowing and understanding emotions is integral to increase your own self-awareness.
3. This is also an ongoing process.
4. The magic lies in knowing when an emotion is healthy or unhealthy.

I still find managing my own emotions very difficult, however, the process I go through in order to acknowledge, listen, reflect and process is a lot quicker. It is 100 per cent fine to express your emotions, and I believe that it's important to start showing and talking about them more often.

Let's use sadness and crying as an example. We all get uncomfortable when we see others crying. Even though this is natural, I have attempted to understand why this is often unsettling to witness. Think about when a child cries, they're not yet able to communicate their emotions, so we console them until they stop. A young child learns the pattern *cry, cuddle, get over it* because it is time to stop. What do we do as adults? Cry and think we have to get over it.

It's not necessarily the emotion we need to be aware of, but our *reaction*. When you are experiencing a strong emotion, think about where you feel it most in your body. What is your body's reaction? What do you then tell yourself in your head about the emotion? You might find that you notice the body's response first because you didn't feel the emotion, or quite likely, have learnt to suppress the emotion. Stress and anxiety are probably two of the most natural emotions we can experience that are so strong and prevalent because our automatic response is to get over emotions quickly because it is not only uncomfortable for us, but it's also uncomfortable for others.

When you ignore these emotions for too long, the body's response becomes more noticeable. When you start to ignore the body's response, this disconnects your body's intuition and wisdom and you start operating on your logical thinking, which is tiring work because you are only accessing part of your true potential. The longer you are disconnected to your body, the more you stay in your comfort zone because you don't feel the additional signs the rest of your body is sending you.

When I first started teaching, I began to lose my voice. I went to doctors and they said it was just because I was learning to talk for long periods of time and sometimes, I would get mild tonsilitis. This would happen quite regularly, so I started to ignore it, continue to work without a voice and 'pushed through it'. After a couple of years, it almost sounded like I was always losing my voice. When I first met my husband, he didn't hear my actual voice for at least a month because it was always croaky. Instead of thinking that something was wrong, I ignored it because the funny thing was, when I was teaching, I was fine, it was after school and on weekends when my voice would go. I thought this was because I was using it during the day and week and so then after work and on weekends it sounded like I overused it. And then it came to the end of my six-week school holiday break. I had not lost my voice all holidays and then all of a sudden before returning to work my voice started to crack again. I had just had 6 weeks of very minimal talking! I booked an appointment with my doctor, who sent me to specialist, who saw that I had nodes developing, who sent me to a speech therapist, who said I used my voice safely.

This is when I did start to question more and look for alternative support. I visited a local naturopath who completely opened my eyes to holistic care and therapy! I did not know about chakras and external body energies and even the body's natural stress response. After working with her for a couple of months, we minimised my stress levels, created a plan of what to do the moment I felt my voice start to change and over time it has significantly reduced. I was supressing how I was feeling (and not speaking my mind) and this caused tension and tightening of my vocal chords, and the additional pressure would cause my voice to break and my throat to get sore. If I did not find this out when I did, I would have seriously hurt myself.

HOW TO START TO RECOGNISE AND FEEL EMOTIONS AGAIN

1. Notice when something makes you feel a particular way. Remember there is no good or bad emotion so you can do this for what you perceive as positive and negative emotions. By doing both, you are bringing awareness to how your body responds and what your reaction is.
2. Stop what you are doing to tune in properly.
3. What can you feel?
4. Where can you feel it?
5. If you would like to take it one step further, can you give it a colour?
6. When have you felt this emotion before?
7. What is your brain's reaction to this emotion?
8. What do you want to do next? (Without doing it.)
9. Breathe. Allow yourself to sit with the emotion.
10. What can you learn from this emotion?

DOING A BODY SCAN

I would love to introduce you to a simple, yet effective, way to connect to your emotions and your body. You can choose different times of the day to connect with your body. I like to do it when I wake up, before I go to bed and during the day when I feel like I haven't had a chance to breathe, or I continue to be triggered by things.

1.   Start by concentrating on your breathing.

2.   Take your breath further and concentrate on breathing in for 4 seconds, hold for 4 seconds, breath out for 4 seconds and then pause for 4 seconds before inhaling again. When I say this aloud for my clients and students it sounds like this: in 2 3 4, hold 2, 3, 4, out 2, 3, 4, pause 2, 3, 4.

3.   Now focus on your toes. Imagine there is an x-ray machine scanning from your toes up towards your head. Allow the x-ray machine to scan slowly.

4.   As the x-ray machine is scanning slowly, check in with yourself by mentally asking, 'How are you feeling?'

5.   Then when you feel like an emotion enters your mind, stop and think about what the emotion is. You might want to think about why, or you might like to just release it. If you choose to release it, you may ask if it is your emotion or someone else's. Just have fun with the response. If it is someone else's then say, 'I return this emotion with love and light'.

6.   Keep moving the x-ray machine up towards your head. Once your body is completely scanned. Do one last declaration of returning the emotion or energy to those it belongs to and then 'call back' your own energy that may have been left with others. Once again, just have a little fun with this. This final declaration is signalling the end of the body scan ritual.

7.   Allow yourself to lay with your eyes closed for a few moments. You may like to imagine white light surrounding you or just focus on your breathing.

HO'OPONOPONO

Ho'oponopono is an ancient prayer used to release unwanted energy and emotions. It is another simple and effective tool you can use, and as an added bonus, no one will notice what you are doing. The first time I tried Ho'oponopono I woke up in the middle of the night with a headache. I had been told by a healer I had visited before that if I felt unwell or 'out of balance' for no reason, I should give this Hawaiian prayer a go. So, I started to recite:

I'm sorry
I love you
Please forgive me
Thank you

The brilliant thing about this prayer is that you can mix up the order in which you say the phrases. The main thing is to apologise, thank, send love and forgive. After I repeated the prayer over and over again, I do not know if my headache subsided, but I do know that I feel asleep quickly, so for me it was a win.

FORGIVENESS

We are our own biggest critics! The majority of our expectations come from ourselves. As a result, a lot of the reasons why we feel the way we feel is because of ourselves. Forgiveness is not forgetting. Forgiveness is the releasing of the attachment of energy and emotion. When we free ourselves from this energy, we are lighter, we are clearer and we feel like we have more energy. There are many forgiveness rituals you can select from the above prayer of Ho'oponopono. You can also journal or write letters. Whatever you choose to do, make it part of your daily rituals to forgive. You might like to include what you would like to forgive in your daily journaling practice. You might like to forgive others from your day or in the past.

During my neurolinguistic programming training (NLP), I learnt a technique called timeline therapy (TM). The theory is based around travelling your timeline and looking down on the situation to collect the learnings. It is also a great therapy to release emotions. I recommend reaching out to a coach or trainer NLP practitioner to investigate this further. You can also do a simple exercise by yourself whilst laying down.

1. Select an emotion you want to release or a situation you want to forgive.
2. Imagine an imaginary timeline that goes back in time and moves forward into the future.
3. Imagine flying above your timeline, back to a time where you felt the first emotion you are focusing on or the situation you would like to forgive.
4. Look down at this event and imagine what it looks like and feels like. Ask yourself what you can learn from this situation.
5. Once you have taken notice of what you can learn, fly back along the timeline and see where other similar situations or emotions present themselves. Once again, collect those learnings too.
6. Before you reach back to the present, repeat the Ho'oponopono prayer.
7. Then take a few more breaths and open your eyes.

We have a lot to gain when we release the energy we hold onto.

Forgiveness allows us to release that energy. Once that energy is released, we have the opportunity to move forward and fill that space with energy that serves us!

Chapter 7

Really Looking After Yourself

In my earlier days of my business, I would suggest to my clients to wake up earlier to dedicate that extra time in the day for themselves. This would work for most of my clients but not all. After speaking at many events, I now encourage women to find time in their day to serve themselves first before they think about serving others.

When I was younger, I can remember my mum staying up late and watching television. I am sure I never saw her actually staying up late, so my memories must be from when I was a teenager or when she would say she was tired in the morning and shouldn't have stayed up late. I didn't think too much of this until I found myself in the same pattern a couple of years ago. I just wanted some time to myself and watching television whilst everyone was in bed was blissful because it was quiet, there were no disruptions (well most of the time), and I was doing something for myself. It was always a good idea at the time but then I would soon regret it when I could not fall asleep straight away, adding another thirty minutes onto my late night and then feeling extra tired the next morning. Even more so, it always seemed that when I did stay up late, one of the kids would wake up in the middle of the night needing me, meaning I not only went to bed late, but it would also be a disrupted sleep. Being one to assess when something is not working well, I recognised that I needed to change something. To work out my 'why' and drive me to change, I created a 'pros and cons' assessment.

Pros:
- I get time by myself.
- I get to do what I want to do.
- The kids are asleep.

Cons:
- I stay up too late.
- I can't get to sleep properly.
- I am at risk of not getting enough sleep.
- I am not doing anything really productive, just watching television.
- I am snappy in the morning.
- I struggle to get out of bed in the morning.

As you can see, my cons outweigh my pros, so it was a habit I wanted to change. It's one thing to identify a change, it's another to actually change it. I recommend focusing on the pros: look at that list and work out how to 'fill' that cup. I was craving alone time, doing something I wanted to do, whilst the kids were safe and occupied. This easily led to me identifying that I just needed some regular time to myself. I turned to my weekly planner and looked at different times of the day where I could do this. I spoke to my support team to look after the kids at various times and I communicated with Ben about how I was struggling to fill this need and if he could help me. This resulted in three different times of the week where I knew I was getting time to myself. At first, I busied myself, booking health and beauty appointments, cleaning the house and doing the washing. That's self-care, right? Nope. Well, they are acts of self-care, but it is not about the act, it is about the intention. I was doing all these things because I felt like I couldn't do them with the kids, or it would make life easier if I got it done without them being home. This did not give me the results I wanted. So, I stopped booking appointments, I left the space empty, and I tuned into what I really needed or wanted to do with that time.

This is how you truly look after yourself. You create the space to be with yourself, you tune in and ask what you need and then you do that. During my workshops I ask participants to list morning, daily and evening rituals. These are the supportive habits you can do on a daily basis to really look after yourself. Instead of just calling them habits, I like to call them rituals. Rituals sound more indulgent!

Unlike generating habits, we are creating space for rituals to occur. So, I recommend looking for habits or regular time slots during the day to insert your ritual. For example, pelvic floor exercises. I love sharing this one at workshops, it gets a good laugh! Every time I stop at a traffic light, I do my pelvic floor exercises. Why? Because when else am I going to have a regular time to do my pelvic floor exercises?! When I watch a television show with advertisements, I do push ups or sit ups or squats. After school every day, I make a platter when I want to sit with the kids and hear about their day. After meetings and workshops, I have a bath. Whatever you want to introduce to your life, think about a regular activity and connect the two. Brushing your teeth is great example of how habits become rituals. When do you brush your teeth? Can you put positive affirmations up on your mirror and read them whilst you are brushing your teeth? There are so many creative ways you can include more positive practices into your day to really look after yourself.

List some rituals you would like to introduce into your morning, day and evening routines below:

- What can you do in the morning to set yourself up for success? What can you do to 'fill your own water tank'?

- What can you do during the day that can bring you to the present moment? How can you stop yourself during the day to focus on your breath?

- What can you do in the evening to ensure you get a good night sleep? New research is saying that we need to be preparing for sleep 3 hours prior! I don't know about you, but that means I am winding down in the afternoon instead of pushing myself to get more done. Or perhaps you are energised at night time. What can you do to ensure that you are using this time (and energy) wisely?

Morning Rituals	Daily Rituals	Evening Rituals

MASLOW'S HIERARCHY OF NEEDS

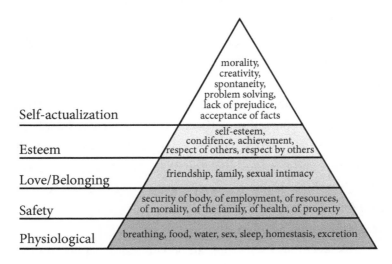

IMAGE: Maslow's Hierarchy of Needs Diagram. Image by J. Finkelstein via
Wikimedia Commons. Used with GNU Free Documentation License.

One of the most eye-opening philosophies I learnt whilst I was studying to be a teacher was Maslow's Hierarchy of Needs. This structure was for students, however, for the purpose of this book I have selected a diagram showcasing the needs of an adult. In order to be at a level where we feel self-fulfilled, we need to satisfy the needs below, as these are our foundations. Now, I don't know about you, but as soon as I read the first layer 'physiological needs' I automatically think, *uh-oh* because I know there have been times where I have not eaten properly, drank enough water, or gotten enough sleep or rest. No wonder I was not feeling my best and it seemed like everything was against me, I wasn't taking care of my basic needs! So, one of the first things you can do more of is include your basic needs in your self-care menu and make them a priority.

Next on the list: security and safety. This one can be a little more complex. Depending on your living, financial or relationship situation, you may or may not feel safe or secure. So, when you have a moment to reflect in your journal, ask yourself, 'Do I feel safe? Do I feel secure?' and see what it brings up for you.

The next stage is what I like to call 'the connection stage'. Connection to yourself and others. Take a moment to look back at 'The Sun' activity in Chapter 2. What did you score yourself in romance and relationships? You might find that you feel good enough in this area that you can progress to the next level or you may find that you need to spend some time strengthening this area before moving onward.

Self-esteem and self-belief are key. It won't happen on the outside unless you change it on the inside. If you are experiencing trouble on the outside, you need to focus on what is happening on the inside. You can review Chapter 5 if you feel the need to strengthen this area.

Once you have worked through these layers and you feel like you have them covered, you reach the self-fulfilment/self-actualisation stage. This is the stage where you feel like you are living your purpose. You are enjoying life, you have time for fun, you have time for hobbies and creativity. When I am feeling like I am not having fun, I know that I am not meeting my needs. I take a moment to look back and start from the beginning. Most of the time, I am not getting enough sleep. Or I need to organise a catch up with a friend or date night with my husband. Sometimes I feel like I am not doing anything right and dropping all my juggling balls. Often I find it is because I am being too hard on myself, and I need to spend some time revisiting my positive affirmations. Once you become familiar with the hierarchy of needs, you can refer back to it when you need to reassess where you are lacking.

It is important to really start looking after yourself. If you don't feel comfortable enough to do it for yourself, do it for others. Remember to lead by example and then inspire those around you to do the same—not by telling them but by showing them.

Chapter 8
Resting and Relaxing

When I first started teaching, I would have weeks where I felt like I was super productive, staying back late and getting all my work tasks completed. The following week, I would get home and sit on the couch, and not move until it started getting dark, and even then, sometimes I would stay put hoping I would get the energy soon to move. I now know that this would have been the result of being in my Autumn Week but at the time I just thought I had run out of energy.

When I first met Ben, this part of me was amplified. Ben is the type of person who will not sit until everything is completed. He would often get home from work and wonder why I hadn't done anything since getting home from work. I never had the words to explain that I just needed a moment to sit and recharge before getting started, whereas his philosophy was, get everything done while you are moving and then relax (or in his case, collapse).

Even on one particular afternoon, I finished work, got home, set the kids up and then said that I needed to have a minute to myself. I allowed myself to go through all the negative thoughts: *you should be playing with the kids, you wanted to exercise straight after work every day this week, you should be getting everything done before Ben gets home*, and so on. And then I just stopped. I asked myself, *what do I really need right now?* I listened, and the answer was rest. So, I did. When Ben got home, he knew that I had been relaxing and he now knows that this means I will be supercharged for the night time routines. And I was.

As humans, we need to rest, relax and have quiet time to connect to our intuition and inner voice. We no longer have to feel guilty for stopping. We can give ourselves permission to stop and just *be*. One great way to do this is to get out into nature. Do you remember what it feels like to be outside at night time? One of the first online programs running through the Lead and Inspire memberships focuses on a lot of what we have spoken about in these Align chapters and specifically encourages you to go outside every night just before bed. This can be as simple as sitting outside. Take a moment to look at the sky. Take a moment to breathe in the air. You might also like to write in your journal or think about what you are grateful for. Like we spoke about in Chapter 7, you may even create a new evening ritual before bed where you go outside barefoot so you can ground and balance, follow it with a journaling session— perhaps even a meditation—and then finish with what makes you grateful.

Other ways you can connect with nature include:
- Walking outside (safely) without shoes on.
- Visit local playgrounds and parks.

- Visit local bush land areas and national parks.
- Go on family adventures.
- Catch up with friends for walks along the coastline.
- Swim at the beach—don't even worry about how cold it is or what you are wearing. Just go all in!
- Dance in the rain.
- Run through the sprinklers again.
- Having your morning coffee, tea or breakfast outside.
- Pat animals.
- Start a veggie garden.
- Do some gardening.
- Introduce indoor plants.
- Have picnics more often—even in your front or back yard.
- Speak to the trees (yes, you read that correctly).
- Make cubby houses with your children.

Basically, there is no right or wrong way to connect with nature. It really is as simple as stopping and going outside. Make it a priority to do more of it.

Do you remember what it actually feels like to relax? You might be surprised by what actually relaxes you. When I was a teenager, I loved waking up later on Sunday morning and doing my homework in front of the television whilst lying on a beanbag watching a 'girly' movie. Guess what I love doing now? Waking up early on a Sunday, spreading all my creative projects and admin paperwork on the theatre room floor and picking at a pile whilst I watch a supernatural series on Netflix. Same, same but different! I used to think sitting down in front of the television after work relaxed me, and there are days where it does, however, quite often I would struggle to get up and then have lots of things to get done (school lunches, dinner prep and the washing, to name a few) then find myself rushing to get everything done before dinner time. So, I took some time to trial different ways to relax after work. When I get home, I change into my active wear, I unpack the school bags, run the dishwasher, make the lunches and prep dinner whilst preparing the after-school snack. If I am really tired, I call someone whilst I am doing it. The kids know to leave me until I have made the after-school snack, and they spend time resting, relaxing or playing outside. We then all eat the snack together. I find if we eat outside on a picnic blanket, I don't worry about what I have to get done inside the house, plus I am connecting with nature. This winds my body and mind down really quickly. If I've had a hectic day at work, I have a shower as soon as I walk in the door. There is something to be said about 'washing the day away'. I still put my active wear on afterwards, or if I really feel the need, it's pyjamas straight away.

Here's the thing, resting and relaxing does not need to be massages and baths. It can be, but they are not the definition of relaxation. You can decide what relaxes you. You might find that a sweaty workout with your favourite music on may be what you need to release the built-up energy and relax after your day. Meditation is often recommended to calm your mind and relax. For me, meditation is less about relaxing and more about connecting to my body and calming my mind so I can think clearly and be productive. Meditation may be relaxing for you.

Use your journal to brainstorm some different ideas for rest. Find what actually relaxes you. The main thing I'd love you to take away from this chapter is to see that resting and relaxation is not lazy but a way to supercharge and amplify.

Chapter 9

Positive Relationships and Your Support Network

Surround yourself with likeminded, positive and loving people and it will make your life much easier! I really make a point of teaching my students to avoid claiming they have 'best friends'. There should be no need to classify friendships as 'best'. We all know that the best does not last. We have 'best before' dates on food. We also have 'best before' dates on our relationships, except we don't know when the exact time is. As we get older, we may think that our friendship circle shrinks because we have less time, our families grow, and our lives get busier. I think it has more to do with the fact that we have had a lot of bad experiences with friendships ending and we don't want to put ourselves through it again. Why would you when you can avoid it altogether? As you would have seen in Maslow's Hierarchy of Needs, connection is an important layer. So, we need to prioritise our relationships and understand the fluidity of all relationships.

When you look back at your past relationships, can you identify the friends that were there for:

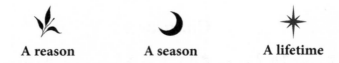

| **A reason** | **A season** | **A lifetime** |

All relationships can end suddenly, negatively or positively. Each relationship can be classified as a reason, season or lifetime. If they were in your life for a reason, they most likely helped you through a stage in your life, or perhaps taught you a lesson (either good or bad) or perhaps you were forced to be friends because of outside factors. If they were there for a season, this may be because of a timeline in your life. You perhaps even thought they were going to be lifetime friends but for some reason you grew apart or it ended abruptly. However, your reason and season relationships ended, please give yourself time to forgive and thank. You may even notice that you have friends in your life at the moment that are there for a reason or a season. Don't think that these are not good relationships, you do not want to avoid these relationships because you feel like the lifetime friends are the ones that matter. Lifetime friends are those who stay with you through all stages of life. They are the friends who you can go a long period of time without speaking and then pick up where you left off the next time you see them. These are the friends you can call in the middle of a crisis even if you can't remember how long it has been since you last spoke.

All types of relationships are important. You never know which category they land in until you start examining the relationships you have. In another online program I run through my membership, we look at doing a relationship audit.

It is an opportunity for you to review your relationships and see if they are bringing the best out in you. You can take a moment to think about how the people make you feel before, during and after you see them. If at any point in time you start to notice a pattern where you do not feel happy or positive, you may need to take some time thinking about how the relationship operates. You do not need to think about throwing the relationship out completely. Instead, reassess your interactions. Do you need to minimise interactions? Do you need to bring different conversations to the catch ups? Just like I asked regarding your pyjamas, how old are they? Do you need to throw some out? Do you need to buy some new ones? Do you even like them? Are they supporting you?

Surround yourself with people who make you want to be a better person. Not because you feel like you are not good enough but because you want to reach your fullest potential. Gravitate towards people who teach you things, who you can learn from. You may find people who are a couple of steps further along than you are in life. You might like to spend time with these people to expand your thinking and perceptions.

If this chapter hits hard for you, revisit Chapter 6 to work through the emotions that are coming up. You may also like to do one of the forgiveness exercises. One of my favourite exercises to do is a 'cord cutting' meditation. You can simply search and find one that you like or follow the simple steps below.

CORD CUTTING EXERCISE
1. Allow yourself to sit or lay comfortably.
2. Take a moment to breathe and just be. Don't worry about deep breaths or trying not to think too much in your head. Just lay or sit for a while.
3. When you feel like you are ready, imagine cords or

'strings of energy' coming out of you. There is not a right or wrong way. Just imagine crazy cords coming out of different parts of your body or even from the same space.

4. As you imagine these cords, think of what colour they are, and make them super bright.
5. Then think of sending love down the cords to whoever they are connected to.
6. Once you feel you have sent enough love, imagine cutting the cords.
7. As you cut the cords, return that love light to you.
8. Imagine or say in your head aloud, 'I call my energy back to me'.
9. Allow yourself to lay or sit with lots of light around you and imagine it warming you inside.

A LITTLE BIT OF WHITE (WELL, COLD) MAGIC

Now this might sound a little crazy to you, but I love a bit of magic and all things spiritual. I came across this little magic trick before I even started my personal development journey. For this activity to work, please have a loving intention. It is with the most love (along with whatever emotion you feel) that you do this activity. This activity for 'removing' people from your lives. Yes, I know that sounds bad and you probably even re-read what I had written. Remember, our intention is full of love. Love for the person to be released from your energy field and love for yourself to no longer have them in your energy field. This does not result in people dying or anything bad happening to them. Instead, it is all about removing the energy that this person expels into your world. You might find that there is a person in your life that you may need to let go of, but you know that you cannot have a conversation or power to make it happen. You might have a friend who you love dearly but is going through a lot at the moment and you can no longer help or support them and feel that it is best that you both move on. You might have family members that make you very nervous before you visit them, making family events very stressful. Whatever it is, you are safe to do this activity and this activity is just as safe for them. Plus, have a little fun with it, you will be surprised the outcome.

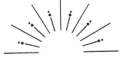

Step One
Write the person's name on a small piece of paper.

Step Two
*Get a small container and put the name/s
in the container.*

Step Three
*Put the container at the back of the freezer
and forget about it.*

Step Four
*Randomly think one day about the person and
the way you used to feel and chuckle to yourself
that this actually worked!*

That's it! I absolutely love this activity. I still surprise myself when I think later down the track, 'I haven't seen *** for a while—it's brilliant! Or there are times I think 'Wow, I don't feel **** anymore when I see ****.'

KNOW YOUR SUPPORT TEAM

Sometimes as busy women we forget that we can ask for help or we can be looked after by others. I think this comes from doing things so well and having control that when we do give the opportunity to someone else, it's not done the way we like it, or our expectations are too high. Instead, we think it's easier to do it by ourselves because we will just have to do it again anyway.

I used to believe that my sheets had to be folded neatly and the kids' clothes drawers must always be organised. What a waste of mental energy! When I first met my husband, I never saw how he folded his sheets, and we didn't live with each other until after we were married because I was teaching in rural Western Australia. The first time I saw him fold sheets, I was shocked. He just rolled them up! At that moment, I thought about something my mum had said to me: if I want help around the house, don't be picky with what you get. So, I thought, the sheets are clean, they are put away and someone else has done the job. No need to worry about that then! When I did the sheets, I still continued to fold them the best I could. I think mainly because of time. Now that I have kids, they get rolled and I think back to the fact that they are clean, they are put away and now even the kids can do the task for me.

Just let it go! Think about what is really important and be intentional with what occupies your mental load. Ask yourself, 'Where are these expectations coming from?' Nine times out of 10 they will be coming from you. So, you can choose which expectations are worth holding onto and which ones are worth releasing.

I remember having discussions at mothers' group about how hard it was to get out of the house and how it felt like we (the mums) were the ones who had to get everything ready because they (the partners) had no idea what to pack or do. This made me think, why don't they know what to do? Do women just instinctively know what to do? Do we set high expectations of our partners and believe that they should do things the way we do things?

So, one Saturday morning, I was flustered running around getting myself ready and Ava and Ben asked if I was ready yet. I was emotional and said, 'Yes, but it is a lot more than just getting myself ready now so I will have to show you how to get her ready too.'

Ben didn't think too much about it, and it wasn't like I organised a lesson or anything, but really, I just started talking to him about what he could do, for example, what to pack in the nappy bag and narrating what I was doing to get ready so he would start to take on the information. Now, there were times where something was forgotten, but you know what? There were times where I forgot things too. The main thing was, I accepted Ben to be on my support team and I communicated how he could help me. This time has rewarded me tenfold because Ben has always been able to take both kids out since they were newborns which has meant that I have had time to myself when I have needed it. You may not have a partner like this, but you will have people on your support team.

Your support team is your network of people around you that can help, are helping or you would like to help. These can be friends, loved ones, family members or service providers. Part of this exercise is identifying who is on your support team, working out what they are on your support team for, utilising their skills and determining how they can reduce your mental load. It is important to communicate with who is on your support team and how they can help you. It is equally important to thank the people on your support team and show gratitude whenever possible. Once you have done this activity you might like to look at whose team you may be on. Who are you providing support to and how can you ensure that the lines of communication are open so you can discuss what to do?

Who is currently on your support team?
How do they support you and how do you communicate with them?
Who would you like to be on your team?
How can they support you and how will you communicate with them?

Once you have identified your support team, think of this team as your own personal squad. You are the coach. How can you ensure your team works efficiently to achieve the desired goal—no grand final here, more like how they can make your life easier! If you have a hairdresser on your support team, you will need to make sure that regular appointments are made in advance and written in your diary. If you have a friend who provides you with support when you need to vent, organise a time to regularly speak with them.

Now let's take it one step further and connect it to what we learnt in Chapter 5. Incremental changes over a long period of time. Did you take a moment to dream and really ask yourself what you would like support with? Did you put down a cleaner, a gardener, a dog walker, a nanny? When I ask this question in workshops, I get so many women saying that they wanted to write it down, but they thought they should take the activity seriously. Oh my goodness! We are even too scared to write down what we really want because we don't think that others will take it seriously. The people you have written on your support team do not have to be on there right now, you can incrementally make the changes and get them onboard when it suits or is available to you. However, I would like to encourage you to trial some people on your support team to see if it does work.

I remember when I first asked if we could get a cleaner. Not only did it take me three months of journaling to justify it to myself and to convince myself that I wasn't failing as a mum or 'housewife', but it also then took two weeks of researching the right person. I explained to Ben why we should hire someone and that my business would pay for it. And then I used to clean before and after the cleaner came so I could keep the cleaner! I laugh at myself now. I slowly started to trust my cleaner—who was on my support team for a reason—and then started to do the work I wanted to do instead of having to clean the house. Then the most magical thing happened, not only did I have time to do my business work, but I also had more time to play with the kids or go on family adventures, and I had more time and energy (and interest) to do those jobs around the house we tend to avoid after cleaning the house, because really, the cleaning never stops! When our budget changed, I opted to stop getting my hair done so I could keep my cleaner. So please, do not think that you are not taking this exercise seriously if you write down people on your support team that you think will never be on there, because that is exactly the whole point.

You are in this exact position because of the resources you have right now.

If you ask for more support or support from different people, then you will be in a different position.

Do not hold back. Establish the best support team possible for yourself. This is all about creating the life you want to live!

We have now come to the end of the ALIGN section of this book. Congratulations! I hope that you have been able to introduce a lot of strategies into your daily life and you feel more connected to who you are and what you want. Please refer to this section regularly to remind you of different strategies you can try out. I have a special group of Lead and Inspire Community members who have been with me from the very beginning. I have now been speaking about the information in this chapter on repeat and to this day they reiterate that they know I have said it before and they know they have done it before, but they still love the reminder of what to focus on. I think this is so important to mention because you do not have to action everything in this book, just select what is relevant to you right now. You can dip in and out whenever you want to. All I want to do is to encourage you to try new things and look for ways to grow. Now let's dive into our natural feminine energy cycles!

Part 2

Know your cycle

Chapter 10

Let's Start with Tracking

Once you have a better understanding of the real you—how you work, what holds you back and what inspires you—it becomes so much easier to be the best version of yourself. In this chapter we have part of a journal which is a tool to help you track your personal cycle in a number of areas, including energy levels, eating patterns and general mood. So, when you feel tired and drained for no obvious reason, you will know why. Instead of wishing for more time and energy, you will have a better understanding of how you work, and then utilise the time and energy you have. Once you are aware of your changing cycles, with a bit of planning, you can ensure your day's itinerary doesn't feel overwhelming and there are tasks that you look forward to. There will be enjoyment, laughter and productivity! It's also important to remember that there's no shame in asking for help. See your friends, family and others as part of your support team: those who will support you to be your best. Please seek professional advice and help at any time you feel you may need it.

UNDERSTANDING CYCLES

We experience cycles every month and by better understanding them, we can better plan for them. Does the following sound familiar: you receive an invitation two weeks before a party and you're so excited to attend, then that weekend arrives and it's now the last thing you feel like doing. Another week you might feel completely in control of everything: the house is sorted, you are on top of things at work and you are so pumped that you make a list of tasks for the following week... only to achieve nothing at all. It's something we all experience, yet we don't stop to ask why. So, let's break it down so you can take control of your cycle, rather than letting it rule you! Your first step is to reconnect with yourself.

Journaling 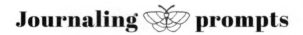 prompts

These are some behavioural questions you will be asking yourself over the course of a cycle:
- What activities do you like to do every week?
- How do your feelings change every week?
- What foods do you crave at different stages of the cycle?
- What are your energy levels from week to week?
- How emotional do you get from week to week?

Challenge the following assumptions:
- When did being busy become something to celebrate?
- Why do we feel like we always need to be doing something and that rest is only something we do when we sleep?

LET US START WITH THE MOON KEY CYCLE

The following image describes the different stages of the moon and how you can possibly feel during this time. The moon has a strong gravitational pull on the Earth and can consequently influence the tides of the ocean. Imagine what this effect can have on your body. I recommend to women that you have a little fun by going outside at night time; just before you go to bed, look up at the sky. Look at the moon and see if you can identify what stage it is. Once you know what stage, you might like to use this image to determine how you are feeling and see if any of the suggestions resonate with you. This is also a great cycle to truly create the life you want to live. I will share this magic with you later on in the book.

You will see, as you follow the cycle, the moon starts off as a new moon, meaning the start of the cycle, just like the start of your menstrual cycle. It is quite interesting to read what women used to do before industrialisation and technology. When life was simpler women would often bleed with the new moon and be sent to tents to all complete their cycles together. They would also take their children but their normal duties that would keep the 'tribe' operating would cease. It would be a time of rest and release. I don't know about you, but I would love to stop all my duties to go to a 'tent' (or a hotel room sounds divine) and just rest, release and set intentions every month. This was a way women could honour their cycles. It was also very common for women to start their menstruation at the same time as others, if not the whole tribe. This is why you might often hear of new moon rituals, workshops and get-togethers.

As the moon moves from new moon to full moon, its visibility enhances. It is energised. This also relates to your cycle because after you have finished menstruating, you start to feel your energy increase. The height of both your energy and the moon's energy is at the full moon. Have you noticed how you feel around the full moon? Do you notice a difference in your children? Or even the people around you? The moon is fully illuminated during this stage, and so are you, fully charged and possibly ready to explode if you are holding onto what you accumulate during every cycle. The full moon can also be connected to ovulation—the release of the egg. The highest peak of fertility and yes, possibly the highest level of unusual behaviour. This is a great time to release emotions and built-up energy you have inside of you, instead of supressing and hiding it with something else like food, drugs, alcohol, gambling, bullying, dangerous and risky behaviour—whatever your vice is.

You may notice in the couple of days before, during and after full moon time, you may not sleep very well or have dreams/nightmares. I often put out a mattress on the floor in our bedroom as it is often the time one (sometimes both) of my children will wake up after having a bad dream. It is a time where we feel more sensitive and intuitive. It can also be a time where we feel reactive and defensive.

After the full moon, the cycle decreases and slowly the moon visibility reduces. This is a sign of the energy dropping, just like you would possibly feel. And then it continues until the new moon again, where you can reassess, reflect and let go before you enter a new cycle.

Now this is the 'traditional' moon cycle, but you might find that you are more closely aligned to the full moon being day one of your cycle, in which the above cycle I explained would be flipped on its head. It is also at this point in time that I point out that this also means that there are women at different stages of their cycle all the time, and around the full moon and new moon you will potentially have a large group of women either menstruating or being highly fertile and at their highest energy. Some at the highest level of energy and confidence and some at the lowest energy and self-belief. Imagine that party!

Take some time to become curious with the moon and how you feel during different times of the moon cycle. You might surprise yourself. I recommend tracking your cycle according with the moon first if you are moving from menstruation to menopause, experiencing menopause, passed menopause, on hormonal replacements, on hormone disrupters, in your fourth trimester or having no idea of your cycle.

MOON CYCLE KEY

We still don't fully understand the effect the moon has on us, just that it does influence behaviours. Learning how the moon changes and then recording your individual experience at these times can be helpful in understanding your personal rhythms.

New Moon	Consider this the beginning of the cycle. The moon is completely black and this is the time to set your intentions for the month ahead. Dream and set goals.
Waxing Crescent	This represents the beginning of new things. It is the growing stage. Build upon the foundations you put in place during your previous cycle or what you set out to do at the new moon phase.
First Quarter	Really make the most of all your energy! Tick off items on your to-do list.

Waxing Gibbous	You may start to feel more emotional than usual. Take a little time to listen to what your body needs – you may need to slow down to make the most of the next wave of energy coming your way.
Full Moon	The midway point of the moon phase. This is your peak time! You may feel extra emotional or charged so utilise this energy in a positive way. You may have been working non-stop until this point and as the moon phases continue it will be time to slow down and assess where you are at.
Waning Gibbous	Time to start finishing projects, crossing things off your list, dropping unimportant tasks and preparing to have some down (or even hibernation) time.
Last Quarter	Begin resting, reflecting and reassessing what you have achieved in the month.
Waning Crescent	Start preparations for the new moon cycle. Roll with the energy you have over the next four weeks! Utilise the time and energy you have to get the activities you feel like doing according to the time of the month.

SEASONAL WEEK KEY

As we progress from looking at the moon, becoming familiar with the moon stages and how we feel during each stage, we start to look at applying the method of 'seasons' to our cycle by grouping 5-7 days together to define a 'week'. In the following image you will see how I have connected the moon stages with a 'season'. Once again, if you are operating the opposite way to how I explained in the Moon Cycle Key section, then you will need to flip the moon stages with their corresponding equivalent.

When you are tracking your cycle, I encourage you to connect to the four seasons: winter, spring, summer and autumn. Day one of your menstrual cycle is the first day of 'winter'. In order to keep tracking as simple as possible in the beginning, I have allocated the typical 7 days to each 'week'. When I refer to a week, it does not necessarily mean that you start on a Monday. You start whatever day you start bleeding. You can then count the days, and knowing that each week has 7 days, you can predict when you will be moving into the next season and stage of your cycle. As you become fluent with your tracking, you will be able to identify when each stage starts and ends, while knowing that some stages have fewer or more days than others. To ensure success, I like to keep it simple by sticking to 7 days.

The moon phases can be described in simpler detail by following the seasons. When you think about the seasons, think about the weather, how you feel, what is happening in nature, how you socialise, what you eat and what activities you do.

NEW MOON AND WAXING CRESCENT

Season
Winter (Days 1-7 of Menstrual Cycle)
Mood
During this time we like to hibernate.
We often stay at home to avoid the colder weather and meals
tend to be warming, slow-cooked and hearty.
Nature
In nature, the rain waters your dry earth.
Animals hibernate and rest for when they need to
venture out in the warmer months.

FIRST QUARTER AND WAXING GIBBOUS

Season
Spring (Days 8-14 of Menstrual Cycle)
Mood
After locking ourselves away for a couple of months we start
to feel like we want to get out of the house and socialise. When
the warmer weather appears, we seem to have more energy.
Spring cleaning is actually a thing because we have been in our
homes for so long we have seen what our habitats contain and
want to sort it all out.
Nature
In nature, new sprouts begin to grow. Flowers begin to
bloom. It is a new beginning as plants have been

dormant and animals have been hibernating.
Time to start feeling the warmth and grow!

FULL MOON AND WANING GIBBOUS

<u>Season</u>
Summer (Days 15-21 of Menstrual Cycle)
<u>Mood</u>
It's warm so we like to get outside and enjoy the weather. It's a time to socialise and we tend to prefer eating lighter food.
<u>Nature</u>
Both animals and plants harness the sunshine but too much can cause problems!

LAST QUARTER AND WANING CRESCENT

<u>Season</u>
Autumn (Days 22-28 of Menstrual Cycle)
<u>Mood</u>
We welcome the cooler weather after the warmer months. We have enjoyed socialising but are now looking forward to spending some time at home and the invitations to outings slow down. Trackie pants and TV anyone?
<u>Nature</u>
The leaves begin to fall off the trees and animals prepare for winter.

Now that you have a little overview, let's begin with the tracking side. The following pages have space for you to write what is happening for your during your cycle. You can choose to start on your day one or right now if you can connect to how much energy you have and the corresponding season. Whichever cycle you are using, start thinking about your personal inclinations and energy levels over the weeks. Refer back to the behavioural questions outlined at the start of this chapter. Remember, 'winter' is the start and is day one. Day one can be the start of your period, the full moon or the new moon. Allow yourself to track over a couple of cycles so you can compare notes. You will find that one month you will identify something and then the following month you will notice something else. Have fun with this process, study yourself, look after yourself, set yourself as a priority.

I have started with what I personally experience before moving onto a guide for you to make general observations. Once you feel confident in your feelings, your energy levels and the tasks you like/don't like to do, you can start using the next planning pages to outline out your week according to your cycle. This will aid you in knowing what works well during your seasonal weeks and what should be switched to another week.

There is no perfect, right or wrong way to track your cycle. It's all about the observations and experimenting. Have some fun with this.

Are you ready to get started? I am so excited for you! Here is an example of what I personally experience so you can be guided in how you can start to articulate what is happening for you each month!

WINTER WEEK

Mood

I feel very strong during this time (however, others may have an experience more similar to my 'autumn'). This is my planning week for everything: I put structures in place because in the next two weeks I will have the energy to get them all done. This is a great time to rest and relax more because in doing so, I will have more energy in the weeks to come.

Planning

I prefer not to speak to people because I want to get tasks organised and completed on my own. It is the best time for me to get 'pen and paper' jobs done. I am more creative and intuitive at this time. I always feel like hearty meals. This is the week I feel like calling people and making appointments for the month.

SPRING WEEK

Mood

This is my most energetic time. I make sure I save all my tasks for the month for this week.

Planning

This is my power week. This week I get the most compliments. I feel like eating well, exercising and socialising.

SUMMER WEEK

Mood

This week I know my energy is starting to run out, so I only try to complete the tasks that need to be done. I allow myself to be okay with not getting everything done because being hard on myself is using energy I'd rather spend on the activities I feel like doing.

Planning

This is the week I like trying new recipes. I still feel like socialising. I get the jobs done that I need to. I feel like healthy meals. Everything feels like it is all balanced and I am handling things really well.

AUTUMN WEEK

Mood

This week the leaves are definitely falling off my tree! I am emotional and sensitive. I allow myself to hibernate, rest and relax. I don't push myself too much when exercising and I allow myself to eat a little off track during this time, because I know I will eat better in the other weeks (so I don't beat myself up about it and just enjoy).

Planning

This week I feel really low on energy. I don't feel like putting in as much effort with my appearance. I cook fast and easy meals. I get pimples, headaches and really want to eat sugar and carbohydrates. I want to get things done but it seems like it takes even longer than usual. So, I schedule a lot of self-care and 'me time' activities during this week.

PLANNING

WINTER WEEK	General observations:	How I feel and my energy level:
	Tasks I enjoy doing or feel like doing:	Tasks I really do not feel like doing during this time:
SPRING WEEK	General observations:	How I feel and my energy level:
	Tasks I enjoy doing or feel like doing:	Tasks I really do not feel like doing during this time:

PLANNING

SUMMER WEEK	General observations:	How I feel and my energy level:
	Tasks I enjoy doing or feel like doing:	Tasks I really do not feel like doing during this time:
AUTUMN WEEK	General observations:	How I feel and my energy level:
	Tasks I enjoy doing or feel like doing:	Tasks I really do not feel like doing during this time:

Week:

MOON CYCLE

ENERGY LEVEL

THINGS TO DO THIS WEEK

DAILY MANTRA

DAILY RITUALS

SEASONAL ACTIVITIES

SWEAT SESSIONS

Seasonal Week:

WHAT THIS MEANS FOR ME

MONDAY	TASK		
TUESDAY	TASK		
WEDNESDAY	TASK		
THURSDAY	TASK		
FRIDAY	TASK		
SATURDAY	TASK		
SUNDAY	TASK		

Chapter 11

Menstrual Cycle Explained: What We Should Be Taught at School

Our menstrual cycle actually starts a lot earlier than we think. Although we do not experience the complete cycle until our pre-teen and teenage years, our bodies get ready for the full process in the early years of primary school. For example, you may find that you started having body image issues when you were 7 or 8 years old, or perhaps you remember having a lot of issues with friends around that time. You may have a daughter who you can relate this to. Why? Because female bodies work in cycles. If you were to track when the disagreement with friends or concern of what others think of them, you would find there would be a pattern the next time it happens Track it enough and you can predict before it happens and therefore encourage them to do something different or perhaps look after themselves before they reach that week.

At around the age of 10 (depending on where you live, what school and what beliefs around girls' health are in that particular area), girls are given growth and development classes, teaching them about puberty. I am always surprised at how few girls actually know what puberty is and how many parents just wait for it to be covered at school. These conversations need to naturally occur at home from an earlier age. Ladies, we need to stop hiding our menstrual cycle from our girls. Instead, we should be leading by example and showing them what we do to look after ourselves at each stage. You may not want to explain the full cycle until they are learning about it, but knowledge is power and the more knowledge they have around the subject the more likely they would feel empowered rather than anxious and worried. You may think school has puberty covered. In actual fact, we can only really go so deep with what we can teach to ensure that we don't go past the cultural beliefs of parents. Sexual education needs to start at home. When we start teaching puberty at school, we begin with looking at how to look after yourself mentally, emotionally and physically. We then move onto the changes in the body starting with the external changes and then the internal changes, which is funny because it is the internal changes that cause the external changes.

What you can do to start teaching and having conversations with your daughter earlier:

- Start to talk about your energy levels. For example, 'This week mum is feeling a little low on energy, so I am looking after myself by slowing down and going to bed earlier.'

- Expose them to your menstruation 'care kit'. Have a box or container where you keep your menstruation products. Ensure this is clean and well organised so then your daughter can see the importance of hygiene and respect around her period as well. You may like to also have a heat pack and other items you use to support yourself. Treat your menstruation care kit as something special and filled with everything you need to look after yourself.
- Discuss the foods you are eating, especially before your period and during.
- Learn about what is actually happening inside of you, do you know why your period happens every month? Do you know what causes it? Do you know what is happening at every stage of your cycle? It is difficult to educate others when we do not know what we are teaching.
- Slow down and have time to observe your daughter. Be available to speak to her about whenever she needs. I encourage setting up a regular communication time from a young age so it becomes normal and almost routine to speak to you.
- Decide on what 'life stories and lessons' you would like to share with your daughter to show her that you experienced the same level of 'confusion' and 'growing pains' as she is going through. Please don't use this point as a way of teaching them to avoid doing what you did, but rather framing it in a sense that you made choices and this is the way it ended up for you.
- Make menstruation an open topic in your household, especially in front of all males so it normalises it.

The complete cycle is a roller coaster of hormones, not only changing us physiologically, but psychologically and emotionally. Here is a table providing an overview of what are the changes and moods of each stage of the cycle.

First Stage - Week One
Normally lasts from day 4 to 8

Name of Cycle:
Menstruation
(Part of the follicular phase)

Seasonal reference:
Winter

Physiology:
Bleeding starts.
This is when the old blood and tissue from the uterus is released through the vagina.
A period lasts for 5 to 6 days on average, however, it can also last up to 8 days.

Psychology:
During this time you may feel extra sensitive. This sensitivity may be shown in strength as well as vulnerability. You may be forgetful and not as motivated as usual. It is easier to feel more negative emotions and harder work to feel positive and happy.

Moods, emotions and energy:
You may feel quite strong one moment and completely emotional the next. Energy is lower at this time as the body has another job to work on. You may prefer to be by yourself and doing tasks that require less energy.

Second Stage - Week Two
Normally lasts from day 7 to 15

Name of Cycle:
Follicular Phase

Seasonal reference:
Spring

Physiology:
This stage is all about the egg!
Your body is getting the ovaries ready to release an egg and the uterus building the lining for the egg.
Your face is more symmetrical during this time. Yep! No joke.

Psychology:
It is easier to be happy and have more of a positive outlook.
You may also feel more feminine, sexy and happier with your body.

Moods, emotions and energy:
You may feel a boost of energy. This is also a time where you feel the need to organise and declutter.

Ovulation can happen anytime between day 12 and 15.
This is when the egg is released. You may experience a couple of days where you feel tired and a little irritable.
Some women can feel the release of the egg and experience cramps.

Third Stage - Week Three
Normally lasts from day 14 to 21

Name of Cycle:
Luteal Phase

Seasonal reference:
Summer

Physiology:
The egg transforms and produces estrogen.
Progesterone increases.
If fertilisation has occurred (firstly, congratulations) then you will move onto a different cycle altogether.

Psychology:
You may notice a 'carefree attitude'.
This can work like either feeling like things don't have to be so serious or perceived as you are starting to feel unmotivated

Moods, emotions and energy:
As a result of an increase in both hormones, you may feel fearless!
As the saying goes. 'What goes up, must come down'.

Fourth Stage - Week Four
Normally lasts from day 21 to 28 or up to 38 days

Name of Cycle:
Secretory Phase
(Part of the luteal phase)

Seasonal reference:
Autumn

Physiology:
If fertilisation has not occurred, there is a drop in progesterone and estrogen—and boy don't we feel the drop!

The lining of the uterus secretes chemicals to either support the fertilisation of the egg or start to break down the lining of the uterus.

This is when you may start to experience premenstrual symptoms such as mood changes, tender breasts, bloating, headaches, breakouts.

Psychology:
This is where you may experience feeling less positive and like life is all too hard.

Moods, emotions and energy:
Drop in energy.
Drop in mood.
Drop in motivation.
Drop in self-esteem.
Drop in confidence.

Rise is feeling guilty.

Rise in feeling not good enough.

A good dose of comparisonitis!

Cravings!

Sugar

Carbs

Salt

Now that we know what is happening during each stage of our cycle and how our physiology then effects our psychology, mood, emotions and energy, what else should we have learnt at school?

25 FAST TIPS FOR YOUR CYCLE

1. Take a mirror and actually have a look at your vulva. So many women who attend my workshops are absolutely shocked when I encourage them to take a look.

2. The complete role of your menstrual cycle is not just to reproduce, while, yes, it may result in that, there is more to it.

3. You can only get pregnant around the time of ovulation. Meaning there is a 'window' of several days before and after ovulation where you are fertile. The unreliable part is knowing when you are ovulating, however, there are many tools you can buy from the chemist that can let you know, tracking apps that can give you an idea, and once you are aligned with your body and tracking like a professional, you will notice

your body's cues that you are ovulating.

4. It is important to go to the toilet after sexual intercourse to prevent a urinary tract infection.

5. You know when you are 'ready' to have sex when you have a strong grasp of who you are, what you believe in and strong reasons for the things you say and do. It is more about personal branding and self-identity than it is age and peer pressure. I would even go as far as saying once you completely know your own menstrual cycle and how you feel at each stage, where you can plan your month from the understanding of what happens for you at each stage.

6. You are the only person who can determine the expectations, rules and beliefs of what sex is, what it is for and your role in it.

7. If you are engaging in sexual activities, it is important to protect yourself from sexually transmitted diseases.

8. If your cycle does not feel right or you are experiencing very strong symptoms, please see a women's health doctor or holistic health practitioner.

9. Show responsibility around contraception. Learn, be educated. Ask lots of questions to lots of people and experts. Don't feel any shame or anxiety around asking.

10. Know the full effects of what contraception does to your body. Give yourself time to track how it changes your moods, emotions and energy.

11. Allow yourself to still experience bleeding. Letting it 'flow' is an important part of your menstrual cycle which we will talk more about in the 'Winter Phase' chapter.

12. There is no need to say to a young girl who has just gotten their first period to congratulate them on being a woman. Most of the time they still don't feel like a woman. Instead, take the time to celebrate looking after yourself.

13. Your body may be capable of creating a baby, but you may not be emotionally ready to have a baby.

14. Becoming a woman requires a lot more than just getting your period.

15. Knowing and understanding your cycle is the most beneficial thing you can do with self-care.

16. All good friends should know your cycle! Yep, you should be able to say to your friends, 'I am in winter' and they know that you just need to be left for a bit.

17. Plan a girls night out when you are all in Spring and Summer Weeks! This will ensure that you will have the most energy and feel like socialising.

18. When you receive an invite, work out what cycle you will be in. If they are in Spring and Summer Weeks, then you know you will have the energy to go. If they are in your Winter or Autumn Week, first decide if it is something you really want to attend and then make sure that it is the only event you have on that week, so you conserve your energy (and motivation) to go.

19. If you are finding your daughter is experiencing difficulties with her friends quite 'regularly', start tracking arguments and fallouts on a separate calendar. You will soon see a pattern and you will be able to speak to your daughter about the weeks where your daughter or her friend/s may be more sensitive and emotional (this goes for both ways where they can be

the 'victim' or the 'offender'.

20. Be aware of when you feel like talking on the phone and responding to texts and when you don't. You know the times where you forget to message back? That is most likely to be in your Autumn Week.

21. Your cycle affects your brain! So tests, exams, interviews and meetings will all be affected by your cycle. Your memory will not be as strong when you are in your lower energy weeks, and you likely won't feel as confident.

22. You know those times you jumble your words or spell them incorrectly when you would normally spell them correctly—hello again autumn week!

23. I nearly had a whole chapter on social media and your cycle. Your cycle will affect your use of social media. In your Winter Week, you are more than likely consume and scroll for hours. In your Spring Week, you may find a minute here and there to watch and be part of it but unless you are commenting and socialising you will find that you will not be on it as much. You will be thinking that you actually don't spend that much time on there as you thought you did because of the amount you consumed the week before. Funny thing is, you may have even said that you really need to get off your phone because you are on it so much in your Winter Week and then naturally didn't use it as much the following week. You may also not be on your phone as much in your Spring Week because you are being productive. If you do a lot of work on your phone, you may spend more time doing the work rather than

aimlessly scrolling. In your Summer Week, you may reach for your phone again to see what everyone is up to and what you have missed out on, BUT then there will come a clear time where the scrolling increases. This is a clear sign that you are heading into autumn. You will start to compare yourself to others. You will start thinking that others are doing better than you, and you will start thinking you need to be like others or do more. This is where I recommend you put the phone down or start looking at your own profiles and celebrating you! See, I told you I could almost write a whole chapter on this one!

24. Your cycle impacts the effect of alcohol on your body! Boy, do I wish I knew this one when I went to parties when I was younger! During your lower energy weeks, you will feel the effect of alcohol more. So, drink less, or better yet, avoid it altogether.

25. In the Lead and Inspire Community I like to refer to decisions as a form of currency (I also refer to time and energy as currency12). You will have more 'decision currency' during your Winter and Summer Weeks. I am not entirely sure why, but my guess is because during winter your body wants to do less, and so you do, but your mind is raring to go. During your Spring Week you are busy being productive that your decision currency runs out pretty quickly (so it's really good to have meals ready to go by the time you get to lunch time). In your Autumn Week, well, do we really have to make decisions?

WHAT IS SHE ENERGY?

It is our natural feminine energy cycle that runs through us. It is a cycle that we go through every 28-35 days. This cycle is repetitive, predictable and our very own superpower. *She Energy* is the knowing the complete self-awareness and ability to utilise your natural feminine energy cycle.

After I had Ava, I felt like I had achieved a pinnacle in my life. I had achieved so much: finished high school and university, established my career, gotten married, bought a home, achieved career advancement, and had my first child. And yet I felt disconnected. It was like I was watching my life through someone else's eyes, or rather watching someone else's life through my own eyes. I was present but I wasn't in the driver in the driver's seat. Having a baby can be overwhelming, and there were times where I wondered how others could do this, but I also found that I had extra time in my head. Those late nights and early mornings, the broken sleep, the feedings, they all gave me space to breathe and think. It is at this point that I want to encourage any mumma who is currently up late or feeding their baby to please put their phone away and turn the TV off because this is where the magic happens! Having the time and space to just think and be allows your intuition to speak to you. If you are not up late feeding, find time during the day or early hours of the morning to sit and be with yourself. Connect to your intuition and inner wisdom by quietening your mind and just having space to be. No meditation required.

When I was going through my teenager years, I was an absolute tornado. I was completely disconnected from my thoughts, actions and feelings. I put this down to the school system, not having clear communication lines with my parents and being totally ruled by my hormones. When I learnt about my menstrual cycle, I was just told about what will happen in terms of physical changes in my body and what to do when I bleed. There is so much more we need to know as young women and pre-teens.

I call for a more comprehensive program for becoming a woman. I am not saying that this needs to be something brought into schools, although there would be benefits, I am pleading for it to happen at home. Starting with ourselves and then passing it onto the girls that we raise. Let's begin with breaking down the supportive structures you can put in place from a young age. The best way to do this is to do them yourself first. I truly believe that girls start their transitions to puberty around the age of 8 years old. So, if we can establish supportive structures at that age can you imagine how easy it will be for them to look after themselves and generate self-awareness at an earlier age?

As you would have seen, the first part of this entire book is all about aligning yourself so you can create the self-awareness to connect with who you are. Now that you are able to start tracking, allow yourself to be curious and aware of what is going on. It might take you a few cycles before you start to notice a pattern, and that is okay. Most of all, I want to encourage you to speak about what you are noticing: talk to your partner, talk to your friends, talk to your family, and when you become confident with your cycle, don't be afraid to speak to your colleagues and even boss about it! When I extend the latter advice at my workshops, it always triggers a reaction, but I firmly believe we should be able to have these open discussions. More on that in the 'Utilise and Flow' section.

Chapter 12
How Does Your Natural Energy Cycle Work?

Let us start at day one. This could be day one of your menstrual cycle or the new moon or full moon. You may even be able to identify day one by simple noticing a bigger drop in energy than usual. Day one signifies the first 'week', which I refer to as your 'Winter Week'. A week is not necessarily 7 days, it could be 4 or 5 days, or even 8. Once you start tracking it you will be able to recognise how long it is. For those of you who are just starting to track and organise your time according to your energy cycle I suggest you start with treating your weeks as 7 days.

Every woman will experience their cycle completely differently. I will provide some examples of what you could possibly experience but please know that your energy cycle is completely unique to you, and it is only through tracking your own cycle that you will begin to understand what you like to do, what you do not like to do, how you can support yourself and how to make the most of your time. Once you get really in tune, you may find you can identify what type of foods you prefer to eat, what your spending habits are, what your relationships are like and what tasks are most likely to flow during each stage.

THE FAQS

What happens if I no longer have a cycle?

You may not have a menstrual cycle, but you still have an energy cycle that you will be able to track.

What happens if I am on the pill?

You will be able to better track your energy cycle because you will be able to follow the numbers. Once again, you will still have a feminine energy cycle that you can track!

I don't think I have a cycle.

That's okay! All you have to do is start noticing. This question is one of the reasons I start my workshops with the information I have at the start of the book in the 'Align' section.

Some of this is making sense and some is not relevant.

Great self-awareness! Not all information is relevant to you. A good learner should listen to all information and then SELECT what is relevant to them at the time. You might find that some information will be relevant at a different time.

How do you know when you change over to the next season?

The more you track and the more you become aware you will know when you change over to the next season because you will either feel the change in the energy or notice that you are doing something that you prefer to do in the next season.

Where do I start tracking?

You may like to re-read the chapter on tracking or just start by journaling and writing down how you feel each day. Food was an easy way for me to start tracking. This may be a good starting point for you too or something else may stand out like sleep, exercise, mood and productivity.

I want to start talking to my partner about all of this, but I am worried that they will think I'm crazy!

Yeah, I get it. Ben must think I am completely bonkers every time I speak to him about something I have learnt (and the endless ideas I have). But I think simply speaking about it is the key. Make it become the norm. When you start scheduling your weeks according to your cycle you will start to notice a difference. Then your partner will start to notice the difference. Then you can start talking about what is making the difference.

What happens if I have a huge meeting during my autumn week?

Reschedule it! Haha, if only. In an ideal world we would be allowed to have 3 (paid) days off work when we have our period and all our meetings scheduled when we are feeling powerful. Seriously! If you have a meeting scheduled during your Autumn Week, be proud that you know that you have to do some serious preparation for this meeting. This will mean, having very little planned for the week. Go to bed early. Be prepared for the meeting a week in advance. Allow yourself to stumble a few words because you know this is probable and then go on with what you have to say (no need to apologise or draw attention to it). Dress to impress; you can wear colourful clothes or jewellery that draws attention away from how you are actually feeling.

Depending on the meeting, get your hair and makeup done if it will make you feel good. I once booked my hair to be done when I was going to a workshop as a participant, I wanted to feel good in the room and not self-conscious; it worked a treat!

KNOWING YOUR SHE ENERGY

Throughout this book I have provided lots of ideas of how I utilise my feminine energy cycle. Let's look at how you can start getting to know yours and then move onto how to utilise it. The first step is generating an awareness and tracking your cycle.

Why are we blocking our cycles? Why do so many of us resent our cycles and think of them as an inconvenience? Why are we so quick to take a pill to prevent unwanted pregnancy that, in addition to causing many physiological side effects, can also block our inner magic and power?

I went on the pill when I was 17 because I thought that was what you did when you had a boyfriend and there was a chance that sex may happen. I remember being embarrassed when asking my doctor and I thought he would want to talk me out of it. But it was completely the opposite, I was told that it was a good idea because I would be able to make my period regular—as if it was something that made my cycle better or it was best for my health. I took my pill with great pride thinking I was doing the best for my body. I never missed a day and didn't skip my period. I didn't realise until years later that my friends would skip the 'pink pills' to keep their period away. I just used them as a way to know when to be prepared. Then years later again I learnt that it wasn't even a real period! What the actual! I had been stopping something so natural inside me for so many years, thinking I was doing good for myself and putting up with the side effects of weight gain, horrible mood changes and feeling totally disconnected to my body. In 2008 I chose to finish my teaching degree up north away from my family and then-boyfriend. As I was going to be away for 10 weeks, I felt like I wanted to give my body a break from being on the pill. Not only did I lose weight over the 10 weeks, my food cravings significantly subsided, my moods became more balanced (although that may be because I was away from said boyfriend) and instead of feeling like I was on the run all the time, I started to notice how one week I had energy and the next I didn't. I didn't know that I was feeling my true cycle then, but what I did know is that I like the clarity of my mind and the feeling in my body, so I chose to not go back on the pill again.

Now, I do feel responsible to mention that I completely understand if you have medical needs to be on the pill or other forms of contraception. I simply encourage you to speak with a natural practitioner to support yourself whilst on the pill/ having hormones in your body or perhaps look at alternatives to your symptoms and birth control. You may not like the fact that it could come down to lifestyle changes, that could be highly drastic, but you are worth it, you deserve your best health and most of all, you deserve to feel and experience the natural energy you have inside of you. For those who follow the spiritual way, imagine a world where all women felt their natural cycles and could access their feminine energy! How would that affect oppression? We would be unstoppable and able to drive collective change in the world.

Once you have looked at the hormone blockers you are taking, and you have made the best decision for you, then you can simply start tracking your cycle according to the 'pink pills', meaning, the first one you take will be day one. For those who have other contraceptive devices, have stopped menstruating, are going through or have been through menopause or have other medical conditions that don't produce a cycle, the good news is you still have a cycle to follow. This is with the moon, or you may like to choose your own one after you start tracking and find a pattern.

For those who have no contraception and have a regular cycle. You simply start tracking on your first day of your period. For those who want to track with the moon cycle you can either start at the new moon or full moon as day one, you will soon see if you are at the beginning or the middle of your cycle. Lastly, if you just want to start tracking and see what is revealed to you, you can just start with a calendar, diary or journal and write down your observations.

I ask the Lead and Inspire Community members to start with writing down how they generally feel. Do you feel like you have high or low energy? What foods did you feel like eating? What were your emotions like? What tasks did you complete with ease and what tasks really repelled you? It is very important to not start analysing at this stage. Just simply write down your observations.

Once you have recorded your observations over a couple of weeks or months, you should start to see patterns in how you were feeling, your energy level and the foods you crave. You may even start to see the activities you preferred and the ones you didn't, however, please don't push to see this just yet as it will start to change as you become more aware of your energy levels. Once you start seeing patterns, you may like to start using a formal way of recording what you find. You can use the digital copies that are bonus inclusions with this book, or you may like to purchase your own tracking journal.

It is at this stage that we start to break down how you feel during each week and what you really feel like doing and what you don't. Once you have a good idea of what you like to eat, do and how your generally feel, you can move onto living with this awareness, knowing that you will have less energy this week so you will support yourself by scheduling fewer tasks to do and more rest and recharging activities.

Then you can move onto totally utilising your energy cycle. What are the specific tasks you prefer to do during each phase? How can you complete these tasks before the due date so they align with your seasonal week? A classic example I give is when you receive an invitation to a party or catch-up. Knowing that you are probably not going to feel like doing it during your Winter and Autumn Weeks eliminates two weeks of possibilities, however, if you know that you are not going to feel like going out, you could always suggest a night in together. Alternatively, I am also hoping that if your friends have read this book, you can open the communication lines and express that you will not be feeling like your vibrant self during that week because you are in autumn, to which your friend replies 'I'll bring the treats' and you opt for a movie so conversation does not have to be a priority. If you have an invitation that you really don't want to go to when you first receive it, check to see when the date lands in your cycle and then decide if you are a yes or a no. During my university years I felt like I was sending so many cancellation messages because when it came to things. I said yes, even if I didn't feel like it when it came around. I wished I knew what I know now because I would have reduced so much anxiety of what to say to RSVP to events. I can now confidently RSVP without any concern and also still say yes to events that I know I will not feel like going to but plan my week so I do look forward to it and have the energy to be my best.

You may also like to start planning your weeks according to your cycle by using my stationery. By zoning into your energy cycle and knowing what you will feel like doing, you will be able to have productive weeks and minimise the energy spent worrying that you didn't do something or pushing for something to be done when in actual fact it will take you only minutes the following week. How many times have you completed a task that normally takes you a couple of minutes but can take three times the amount of time on a different week? Or perhaps you spend so much time wishing you didn't have to do it and then do it and wish you started it earlier because it really wasn't that bad. No wonder we are feeling all over the place and burnt out. Our brains love patterns, and it is continually trying to follow the direction of where you are sending your thoughts. If you could align your thoughts with how your body was feeling, how beneficial do you think that would be?

The next 4 chapters are snapshots of my seasonal weeks. Remember that everyone's cycle is different to others and what I feel like doing (or not doing) in my seasonal weeks may be different to yours.

Chapter 13

The Winter Week

LET'S LOOK AT THE ACTUAL SEASON OF WINTER

Winter is often cold and darker. Some areas may experience snow or ice and others may just experience rain. Animals find ways to adapt to survive in the colder months or they may hibernate. Winter is all about keeping warm. Eating warm and nourishing meals and often cooking meat for longer periods of time and using the fruits and vegetables we can access. After a busy summer period we look forward to winter where life seems to slow down and invites tend to wane because the weather seems to keep people at home more. The rain and darker weather can affect people's moods and it appears to take a lot more effort to wake up in the morning, especially if it's still dark!

My Winter Week snapshot

Energy Level	Mood	Food
Mid-level to low.	Fierce to begin with, then extra sensitive.	Warm meals. Easy to prepare and cook.

Movement		Money
Very little.		I have no interest in spending money because I have no interest in going out and do not feel good in my body, so I do not want to buy clothes during this time.

Day 1

When I was younger, my first day of my period was an inconvenience and I felt disgusting. However, if I was playing a netball game, I knew that it would be one of my best games. On the first day of my period, I am fierce and strong during the day. This energy doesn't seem to last long and by the evening all I want to do is eat and watch television. I will want to stay up late, but I know it is best to go to bed early. I find it harder to get up in the morning during my winter week, so I set my alarm 30 minutes later. On my first day I like to celebrate and reward myself. I clear the day of my appointments (if possible) and I allow myself to have a day of pottering. I allow myself to eat sweet treats and enjoy them totally guilt-free. There is always a nice dessert that I look forward to—nothing rushed, something really high quality.

Day 2

Day 2 is my most difficult day of my whole cycle. I prefer to wear comfortable clothes and avoid doing much. I feel low on energy and you can tell it on my face. It takes a lot of effort to boost how I am feeling, and I need to make sure I am prepared to go to the toilet a lot as it is my heaviest flow day. I forget about what I have to accomplish on my to-do list, and because of this, I will often not schedule much during the first three days of my period. I look forward to these first couple of days because I used to always wish for some time off, now I have a couple of days every month where I completely switch off. You may not think it is possible, but when everything else is allocated in their seasonal weeks and you have prepared for these first 2-3 days, your household can run on autopilot and you can really enjoy resting.

Day 3 to 5

I am still low on energy during these days, however, I start to use this time for my allocated winter week activities. When it comes to work, I like to type, write, get reports done, do administration work and work behind the scenes. It is during this behind the scenes work that I set my intentions for the month ahead. What would I like to achieve, what tasks would I like to get done and I start my to-do list for my spring week. At work, this is not the best time for me to have meetings or exert a lot of energy. So, I plan for the meetings to happen the following week and I schedule independent tasks or do paper-based tasks. I also book important appointments for my summer week. I prefer to do tasks that require more mental energy rather than physical.

As discussed before, the Winter Week feels very much like the season itself. If you were to think about the things you like to do in the actual winter season can you make links to how you feel during your Winter Week? For me I love eating roasts, slow cooked meals and warm foods. I also like meals that I can put in the oven and allow them to do their thing. I prefer to wear comfortable clothes and watch television. This is the perfect time to binge a television series or watch some movies I've wanted to make time for.

When it comes to being a mum and a partner, I enjoy doing quiet activities and those that don't require much energy. This tends to be the week where I do writing, drawing, colouring and small art activities. We do more reading together and I will often sit and watch at the playground when the kids play rather than getting directly involved. This used to really trigger my mum guilt because I was comparing myself to how I felt the previous two weeks where I was happy to play and be an involved mum. As a partner, this is definitely my week where I want to be alone. Rather than showing my distance I ensure I do a lot of small gestures to show my love.

When it comes to exercise, I really don't feel like exercising, even walking seems to be an effort, but I will kindly push myself to do it as I know I feel better for it afterwards. This is definitely the week where I am kinder to myself and really make sure I am filling my cup for the month ahead. I once read that if you were to look after yourself more and allow yourself to rest during your Winter Week, you will have more energy for the rest of the month. I am not entirely sure of this just yet, however, I do love resting and watching television without feeling guilty because these are the activities that I prefer to do during my cycle, so I allocate these tasks to this week. As I have spent time planning the tasks I want to do when my surge of energy comes, there is no guilt for not being so productive and I can focus on time for the things that really fill my cup. Listening to podcasts, reading one of the books on my to-read pile, having baths, booking beauty appointments (once my period has actually finished but I am still in the last couple of days of my cycle) all find their place in my Winter Week and as soon as I've enjoyed these activities, I no longer felt guilty or bad when I don't do these things on a regular basis.

It is also during this time that I feel like I am connected to my intuition more. I have this inner wisdom that I can tap into. During my autumn week I feel like a lot of ideas and thoughts emerge, which is why I like to write and journal more in that time. My Winter Week is the week where I tap into a little more of my masculine energy and discern the ideas. This allows me to create a clear plan for the month ahead. Knowing that I am allocating tasks that require the most energy in my Spring Week and the tasks that require socialising in the Summer Week I always make sure I am looking ahead for things that will need to be done according to deadlines. I understand that there will be times where tasks pop up or come out of nowhere, however, because I have allocated tasks in the correct energy cycle they are completed with more ease and therefore quicker leaving extra time for those tasks that were not foreseen in my Winter Week.

Day 6 to 7

I know when my energy cycle is going to switch to my Spring Week when I start to get frustrated with having low energy and I am mentally ready to action my to-do list. I no longer look forward to watching television and I want to get started with my healthy eating and exercising again. It is at this time that I can go to bed earlier and set my alarm for earlier as I will start to wake feeling more energised.

WINTER WEEK SUMMARY:

- Clear my plans for 3 days so I can rest and choose to do nothing.
- I do something to celebrate the start of my period.
- This is a time where I get a chance to watch television (so I do not spend mental energy thinking about doing this during the other weeks).
- I like to do all things self-care in this time.
- I prefer to do tasks 'behind' the scenes and write to-do lists for the rest of the month.
- I set intentions for what I want to achieve during the month ahead.
- I have easily prepared meals to eat.
- I do less with my kids and husband but ensure I do the quieter activities with them.
- I am more sensitive this week and prefer not to have meetings.
- I stay off social media because I can find myself scrolling for hours if I do use it.
- I stay away from alcohol—it just goes straight to my head.
- If I rest and recharge now, I am saving energy for the rest of the month (fingers crossed).
- My Winter Week is no longer a week of inconvenience, I use it as a week to create a steady foundation for the month to come and lay on the self-care heavily—it is divine to be a woman!

Chapter 14

The Spring Week

LET'S LOOK AT THE ACTUAL SEASON OF SPRING

Spring is all about new growth. Seeds can be planted in autumn to receive rain, but spring is the time where the growth begins. You can also seed during spring for new growth in summer. The weather becomes warmer, and it can be wetter. Animals return from hibernation and newborns will also emerge. As humans, we are craving the warmer weather after spending time inside or after having enough of the rain, snow and cold weather. We may also be craving connection and socialising because we have enjoyed the alone time whilst we also 'hibernated'. The term 'spring cleaning' may have come about because we had spent so much time at home, and we saw what we had behind closed doors or perhaps it was because the weather was warmer and we wanted a fresh start to the new season. As the days last longer, projects may be started or planned. Spring is the preparation time for summer break. There is a rush of new energy with the warmer weather and there is something about the warmth that can spring (see what I did there?) you into action!

My Spring Week snapshot

Energy Level	Mood	Food
High	I love life!	Super healthy and light

Movement	Money
Bring it on! Smash it out!	I don't have time to spend money unless it is to do with actioning my to-do list.

Oh, I love my Spring Week. I love the energy. I love ticking things off my to-do list. I love that I feel my true self during my Spring Week. It is during this week that I can do ALL the things, so I make sure I really appreciate and acknowledge myself.

On my first day of my Spring Week, I hit the ground running and start the tasks strategically set out on my to-do list. I feel so productive, and I action tasks very quickly, however, there are certain tasks that I do not action quickly and I know that it is best for me to not do them in this time. Paperwork and writing are definitely not my forte during this week. It is all about doing tasks that require physical energy. I can become easily frustrated if I am not doing tasks that I feel like doing or find that people are slowing me down. If meetings are scheduled and do not have a specific agenda, I definitely become irritated so it is important for me to recognise when a task or meeting with very little direction is going to happen so I can see it as way to recharge for my tasks afterwards, otherwise I am just using my high energy on being angry.

The other thing I need to be aware of is that my high energy can be triggering to others who are low. Just like when I am low and I see other amazing women in their element during their Spring Week, I automatically start analysing and comparing myself. I now stop myself from doing this, but I know that others do not have this awareness yet. I can easily recognise when someone else is on the opposite cycle to me, so when I have more energy, I like to use it to 'boost' those who are not feeling the same way. Small gestures can go a long way, remember they may not be in the mood to talk so little notes and gifts can be enough to make them smile.

It is during this time that I feel the most beautiful. I once read that even our face is more symmetrical during this stage of our menstrual cycle. As a result, I use this time to do the tasks that require myself to be seen. This may mean meetings, recording videos or booking speaking events during this week.

I want to do quick tasks with the kids where I feel like I am being a 'good mum' and the kids appreciate the time that I am spending with them. I often pull activities from my 'mum file', those that I have seen on social media, online or in person. Rather than feeling like I should be doing these types of activities all the time, I do them when I have the most energy to do them. That way I am doing them at least 12 times a year!

Food during this time is quick and light. I love eating healthy and nourishing my body and it is during my Spring Week where it is so much easier to stick to a plan or make healthier decisions. During my Spring Week, it is common for me to open up my pantry or a kitchen cupboard, clean it out and reorganise it! The fridge also gets a wipe out and when I go through each room in the morning and evening, I sort things out. It is 'spring cleaning' in action every month!

It is towards the end of my Spring Week where I like to be social. I put it down to the fact that I am about to enter my Summer Week and because I used a lot of energy getting tasks done that my body naturally wants to do something different. And because I feel good about the way I look it is nice to go out. This is the best time for me to go clothes shopping as I am happy with my body, and I am more likely to buy colourful clothes. I highly recommend you organise shopping sprees during your Spring Week so you do not buy on impulse, rather you buy what looks good, as a result you end up with a wardrobe you would wear in spring! Have a lot of black and dark clothes in your wardrobe? You might look at not shopping during your Winter Week.

Now it might sound like my Spring Week is all sunshine and flowers—and it mostly is—but sometimes I don't feel so energetic during my Spring Week. When this happens, I think about where my energy wants to go. Where I want my energy to go and where it wants to go can be two different things. I would have scheduled so many tasks in this week in the hope that I will have energy to get them done and then sometimes I get hit with a Spring Week where I really don't feel like completely any of the tasks on my to-do list. This is the point where I reach for my journal and I connect with my intuition; I ask myself where I want to focus my energy. Most of the time it has to do with things outside of the office and even outside of the house. As soon as I focus my energy on different types of tasks, I then start to feel energised again. I leave the tasks I have scheduled for my Summer Week (because that is where the 'leftover' tasks get completed anyway) and I enjoy my spring energy doing something different this month.

SPRING WEEK SUMMARY

- This is my highest energy week and therefore my most productive.
- Because I wrote my to-do list in my Winter Week, I am very prepared for all this energy.
- I will often randomly clean cupboards and drawers during this week.
- I feel like completing all the educational and fun activities with my kids.
- I have more energy throughout the day and night so I will be able to get up earlier and stay up later.
- My time is spent on doing tasks rather than watching television.
- This is the week I will cook new recipes and trial new health kicks.
- I feel good and look my best.
- Towards the end of my Spring Week, I like to socialise.
- I don't tend to book appointments during this week because I get frustrated with the time I waste getting to and from, plus the waiting in between. I feel like my time is best spent elsewhere.
- There are occasionally Spring Weeks where I do not feel as high energy and getting my tasks done on my to-do list, so I will tune into where my

energy wants to go and do something different instead.

Days 12 to 15

It is around Day 13 and 14 when I ovulate. It is like a couple of days in the middle of my cycle where I feel a little tired and moody. I know straight away that this is because of my hormones and the egg releasing. And because I know this, I know that I am fertile, and I also know that I feel extra sexy, magnetic and unstoppable. So, I use this feeling to really amplify something. Whether it is my relationship with Ben or a work task—I utilise this spring/summer energy! Think of it like New Year's Eve. It is the time between celebrating Christmas and welcoming in the New Year, how much fun is it and how good does everything feel? Ovulation is quite similar to that, even with the couple of tired and 'rocky' days.

Chapter 15
The Summer Week

LET'S LOOK AT THE ACTUAL SEASON OF SUMMER

Bring on that warmer weather! It is a time of celebration and reaping the rewards of the crops from spring! It is a time to enjoy the warmer weather and get outside and connect with others. The days are longer and there is so much to do. It is easy to run out of time during the day because you have spent so much time enjoying yourself that you forget what the time is!

My Summer Week is all about finalising the tasks I started in my Spring Week. This is the time that I look at what I had hoped to achieve in my Winter Week and decide what is of the highest priority. The tasks that are not of the highest priority are then moved to the following Spring Week. Just note, it is important to recognise if this task continually gets moved to the following month. You can choose to complete it as the first priority next cycle or assess whether it can be dropped completely.

My Summer Week snapshot

Energy Level	Mood	Food
High and then descreasing.	Do I really have to do that?	Super healthy and starting to get bigger/ heavier.

Movement		Money	
Bring it on! Smash it out!		I love spending money on others and food during this time. I have to be careful of going out too much and visiting cafés and restaurants. If I go to the shops, I have to be focused on what I want to buy because I will come out with a lot of things for the kids.	

I am so aware that my energy drops significantly in this week, so I like to get the tasks completed earlier in the week and then have the remaining time for socialising and going to appointments. As mentioned in my Winter Week, I spent time booking the appointments in advance so now all I have to do is go to them. I find it best to do them in my Summer Week because I want to get things done in my Spring Week and I already feel so busy, so I don't want to put pressure on myself by having a lot of tasks as well as appointments.

I can also tell that I am in my Summer Week when I start

running late for things. It is because I am still riding the 'productive' high and getting lots of things done that I decide to do too many things at once like putting the washing machine on 40 minutes before I have to leave, and it is a 45-minute cycle. Not only do I lose 5 minutes with the cycle, but I am also pushing for time as I have to hang it out! *Just leave the washing for when you are home, Jessica!*

I always wonder if I don't feel like doing work in my office because I have spent the last two weeks completing tasks or if it genuinely because my summer energy wants me to get out and about. Think about the actual summer season, when the warmer weather starts and we want to go and see our friends and visit new places. So, this is the perfect week for me to organise extra special adventures and after school trips with the kids. This is the week (well weekend) where I schedule date night, or sometimes the weekend before my Summer Week kicks in because I have a higher libido. Instead of looking at all the places I wish I could go to when I have time, I select these places to actually go to off my list! It is a great time for family holidays or weekend getaways because I have spent time getting things done and now, I can have more fun.

Fun is my focus during my Summer Week! If I asked my kids which week would be their favourite, they would probably say this week too! I play in the playroom, I play outside, I play at the playground, and I run around! Remember our weeks don't always run from Monday to Sunday so this energy can go over two calendar weeks. This is important to remember because it can possibly feel like you are really hitting some high 'mum' goals and then the following week you start to crash in energy and wonder why you are not doing all the things you were doing last week or the day before! The change in energy can be very sudden.

Towards the end of my Summer Week, I can notice the change in energy. I used to—and occasionally still do—feel sad because I know my energy is going to drop and I am not going to be 'high on life' for the next couple of weeks. Although I am starting to acknowledge and be grateful for my lower energy weeks. It is at this point where I clear my to-do list. I follow the Do, Delete, Delegate or Delay method to clear my schedule. This is in preparation for my Autumn Week, so I do not feel overwhelmed with what I have to get done. I want to ensure that only the tasks of the highest priority are on my list when I have less energy so I do not use any energy thinking about all the things I 'wish' I could do. There is no point having things on your list when your energy is not aligned to doing them. All you are doing is wasting your energy thinking about it or feeling guilty about not doing it. Allocate the task to the correct seasonal week where your energy aligns with it and then focus on what the highest priority tasks are.

Exercise is an interesting one during my Summer Week. I get bored easily and require different types of exercise to keep me motivated. This is important because if I am bored, I will not do it and I know it is important for me to exercise in my Summer Week because if I don't keep that momentum going in my Autumn Week (and since I do very little in my Winter Week), I will have some months where I am only getting a good exercise session in my Spring Week. When you think about it that way, I am only going to get 3 to 5 good sessions in a month, which is not enough. So, when you are looking at exercise and your cycle, work out what types of exercise you prefer to do. You may have to change the types of classes according to your cycle to ensure you are getting enough exercise. This used to frustrate me because I would be so strong in my Spring Week and then lose my 'strength' very quickly. I now know that I have to switch it up each week according to my cycle.

As I mentioned before, you may like to have a list going for places you would like to visit or perhaps the family adventures you would like to go on so you can select one of these during your Summer Week. Once I set this system up, I no longer looked at what others were doing and wishing that I could do it too, I started to do the things I wanted to do!

SUMMER WEEK SUMMARY:

- I know my energy is dropping so it is important for me to finish off the tasks I did not get done in my Spring Week and go through my list to determine what is actually a high priority.
- I no longer want to be in my office, I want to get out and about! So, this is a great week for family adventures and getaways.
- Date night for the win!
- I am at risk of running late for appointments, so I try not to do too much.
- My appointments have been booked for this week, so I am still getting things done without too much thinking.
- I love to have fun and play during this time.
- It is a good week to catch up with friends and socialise.
- I need to be careful when I am at the shops

because I am likely to buy things for my family that they probably don't need. So, on the plus side, this is a great time to buy presents for the upcoming birthdays!

- I get bored easily.
- It is important for me to switch up my exercise and to keep doing it!

Chapter 16
The Autumn Week

LET'S LOOK AT THE ACTUAL SEASON OF AUTUMN

Autumn is a time where we start to wind down after a busy summer period. The cooler weather can often be a nice change and earlier days can mean earlier bedtimes. Animals start to prepare for the cooler weather, storing food or travelling to regions with warmer climates. Leaves on the trees start to change colour and fall. Nature itself is preparing for the colder months where growth slows or becomes dormant.

I have had a love/hate relationship with Autumn Week. Even as I write this, I know that it is more of a 'hate' relationship, and I am really working on loving it or at least liking it. I have mostly looked at my Autumn Week as a week where all my momentum stops. It is the week where I am reminded that I am not a superhuman and I have limitations. After firing on all cylinders for two and half weeks, I am hit with an energy drop that frustrates me. Slowing down is uncomfortable for me. I like to be busy. I like to achieve. I love ticking things off my to-do list. This is my comfort zone, and my Autumn Week is yet to feel comfortable.

My Autumn Week snapshot

Energy Level	Mood	Food
Low.	I am easily frustrated and highly sensitive. I am critical of myself.	All. The. 'Bad'. Stuff.

Movement	Money
Although I do not feel like it, movement is really important, so I make sure I at least walk.	This is the time where I want to spend money. It is more like emotional spending rather than emotional eating. I try to avoid looking at online shopping during this time because my will power is very low.

So, what do I like to do during my Autumn Week? My head wants to keep going but my body wants to stop, so it is important for me to align both by closing down my to-do list and know that I will revisit it in my Winter Week where I will organise it again. By closing down my to-do list, it slows my mind because I relax into the feeling that I don't have many things to do. My body wants to rest but it is not at the stage where it wants to do nothing at all, so I direct my energy to being outside with the kids. I may not join in, but I will watch, laugh, tickle and cuddle. This is the quickest way for me to get into the zone of appreciation.

It has taken a long time for me to realise that Autumn Week is all about gratitude, appreciate and reflection. I also feel like it is a time for me to honour my feminine energy more as I have been operating in my masculine energy for so long. If I want to enjoy my Autumn Week and still feel like I am in flow, I support myself by getting better situated in the present and grounding myself. I often know I am in my Autumn Week when my scrolling on social media becomes more like comparing myself to others and yearning for more in my own life. I get off social media in my Autumn Week. I then reach for my journal and start a guided meditation.

I would ideally like to meditate more but during this season I find that I meditate more during my Autumn Week. Remember our definition of consistency can be what we want it to be. I would like to consistently meditate and read... do I do this every day? No. One activity I do in my Autumn Week and the other I do in my Winter Week.

Journaling and meditating really help me to calm my whole system down. This brings me to a clear state of mind where I can reflect on what my month has been like so far. What worked well? What do I want to do more of? What do I want to do less of? Allowing time to reflect and see where I am according to my goals really harnesses the energy for creating the life I want to live. This is the time where I refocus and align back to my goals and visions.

The time I spend with Ben and the kids is at a slower pace.

There are lots of cuddles and talking about our family and values. This is the time where I find myself looking for the teachable moments and times where I will remind my family how much I love them. Ben will cook more during my Autumn Week, and I will spend more time doing slower activities like sitting outside, breathing, journaling, having baths, anything really to slow my mind.

At work, I will start to hibernate (more than I already do) because I prefer not to socialise and want to conserve my energy for my priorities. The leaves are really falling off the trees. My skin changes colour, I have a breakout on my chin, and I feel really bloated. I can choose to wear comfortable clothes or bring my A-game by wearing colourful dresses. This becomes a self-conscious cycle because I am not really feeling good about myself, and I want to eat to make myself feel better. With this awareness now, I give myself permission to enjoy those treats but make sure they count. This also supports me to eat relatively healthy during my other seasonal weeks because I know that this is the week where I emotionally crave more.

The only work tasks I prefer to do is cleaning out. I clean out my emails and messages. It is the time where I unsubscribe to emails that I no longer find value in or are filling up my inbox. I also like to give reviews and leave testimonials. My Autumn Week is a great week to leave love notes to others, hand out thank you cards and really acknowledge the people in my life. Imagine if we all did this every month!

When I start to experience premenstrual symptoms, I make sure I am ready to stop. I also know that there will be a sudden surge of energy, anywhere between 12 to 24 hours, kind of like the last day to get as many acorns for our hibernation time. I like to whizz around the house, put all my work tasks away and make sure everything is tidied away as much as it can be.

AUTUMN WEEK SUMMARY:
- I have a love/hate relationship with my Autumn Week.
- The drop in energy can be frustrating.
- My mind is running fast but my body is moving slow, and it is important for me to ground myself and slow down.
- This is the time for me to tap into my feminine energy more.
- Going outside, cuddles, and all things love and beauty are perfect for this time.
- It is the week for appreciation, gratitude and reflection.
- Work tasks are put on the 'back burner', and I use my energy to clean out emails and messages.
- It is a lovely time to send thank you messages, testimonials and reviews.
- Although I may not like my Autumn Week as much as the other weeks, I still appreciate it because it is signalling to me that it is important to slow down regularly.

I hope my summaries have been helpful as you track your own cycle. Please remember that these are only guides. Every cycle is different and how you feel will be different. We will be moving onto how to utilise your cycle in the next section of the book. This is a game changer!

Part 3

Utilise and Flow

Chapter 17

Feminine and Masculine Energy

No matter what gender you identify with, you have both feminine and masculine energy. The definition of what 'feminine' and 'masculine' mean has been lost over time. We often believe that females are feminine and males are masculine. So, what if we were to create a new understanding of feminine and masculine energy?

In order to feel like we are in flow, we need to have a 'balance' that works for us. You may remember me saying in earlier chapters that the word 'balance' does not mean 50/50 or equal. Only you can determine your balance. When I am explaining what flow means in workshops, I use the analogy of 'pushing a boulder up a hill'. You know the weeks or the tasks that just feel like everything is going wrong, things appear harder than they need to be or perhaps you are working on something that is taking you longer than usual. These are the times where you are not in 'flow' and because of that, your energy is not working for you. Now that you have built your self-awareness you can identify when your energy is not in alignment and when you should select a different task or perhaps a strategy to re-energise you. You may even decide that the task is best left for now and you will come back to it when you know that you have the right energy for it.

I would like to mention at this point of the book that it's important to recognise when perfectionism returns and procrastination becomes a strategy to avoid what is a high priority. If you find yourself avoiding tasks that are of high priority, be honest with yourself and either seek the help you need or allocate the time and space to get the task done.

Knowing when you are in flow increases your productivity and reduces the feeling of angst. Tasks will appear easier, and you will be more efficient and productive with your time. Tasks take as long as the space you allocate to it. How often do you leave things to the last minute or finish them just before they are due? Tasks will always be completed before they are due because the time it is due is often the amount of space you give a task. For example, if you have a deadline and make an agreement with yourself that you will get the task done earlier than the deadline, you may start off strong but then leave the task for a while only to complete it just in time for the deadline. You may even set a new deadline for yourself only to leave it again until the last minute because you knew deep down you still had more time.

I like to break the deadline into smaller 'time-tasks'. When I have reports due, I work my way backwards from the due date. I also calculate where I will be in my cycle and allocate them to the weeks on the calendar. I then break down the final task—

reports being completed—into sub-tasks and then assign them to my seasonal weeks. I take into consideration my energy cycle and make sure what the task requires will align with my energy cycle, for example, I am not going to allocate the major writing part in my Autumn Week where my energy and motivation are low. I allocate the writing part in my Winter Week where I like to work behind the scenes and type on my laptop. Giving myself 'time-tasks' allows me to create smaller pockets of time where I can get the task completed rather than having a bigger task that has a bigger allocation of time only to put it off until the due date and feel extra pressure with getting it done. We no longer have to feel this way. We can be in control of our time. With the knowledge of our own feminine energy cycle, we can really utilise the energy we have, work in flow and create the feeling of having more time and energy!

WHAT IS MASCULINE ENERGY?

We live in a society that is pulsating with masculine energy. I would even like to say that our society wants us to favour the masculine energy and ignore our feminine energy. The result: burnout, anxiety, unworthiness, and feeling overwhelmed and disconnected. Any of them sound familiar? Masculine energy is all about boundaries, restraints, structures, productivity, efficiency, action, busyness, due dates, deadlines and generally do-do-do-do. You can think of masculine energy with your own understanding of what the collective societal beliefs are of 'men': strong, dominant, protector, hunter, provider, breadwinner, powerful, leader, stable, safe, and so on. I would like to acknowledge here that I do not believe these to be accurate because all genders can harness these traits.

WHAT IS FEMININE ENERGY?

Flow. Beauty. Softness. Nurturing. When you think of feminine energy, think of calm, peace, rest, relaxation, pleasure, indulgence, nourishment, slow, heart-warming, love, gentle, and so on. Feminine energy can also bring fire, intensity, strength and power just like the masculine, but in its own way.

Together both energies dance.
Together they both sing.
Together they both flow.
Together they both feel energised.

When you tap into both energies you bring a different level of balance into your life. You may use your masculine energy to set boundaries, create structures and decide on consistent* habits. Then your feminine energy can be used to bring joy, pleasure, rest and calm into your life. You can be just as productive but with a kindness towards yourself and others. Time slows down when you are in flow.

Our masculine energy supports our feminine energy by creating supportive structures. Our feminine energy supports our masculine energy by nourishing, nurturing and recharging so we can continue to DO.

*Remember consistency is another word that you can create your own definition for.

HOW TO UTILISE BOTH MASCULINE AND FEMININE ENERGY

1. Be able to recognise what type of energy feels like to you.

2. Think about which energy you are surrounded by the most.

3. Think about which energy you think you operate in the most.

4. Think about which energy you would like to tap into more.

5. Think about what you can introduce to your life to create more of the energy you feel you tap into the least.

HOW TO CREATE MORE FEMININE OR MASCULINE ENERGY IN YOUR LIFE

Feminine Energy	Masculine Energy
Add more beauty to your home or surround yourself with beautiful things.	Get a calendar or planner that works for you and your family. Commit to using it on a daily basis to create organisational structures in your life. Explain to those around you what the system means and how they can fit into it.
Select clothes that make you feel more feminine.	Select more clothes that make you feel more masculine. If I want to get more jobs done at work, I put my running shoes on; these may not be the most professional shoes, but they make me feel productive so I can tap into my masculine energy.

What makes you feel like you are 'flowing'? To me, it is a maxi dress. Bright, colourful and flowing. When I wear a fantastic maxi dress, I feel feminine.	Look at where you need to set new boundaries and have difficulty conversations.
Up your self-care; nothing screams feminine more than a bath, bubbles, a candle, your drink of choice and quiet time.	Lists. Lots of list. Lists of everything you want in your life.
Going outside more and connecting with nature.	Time-block your day. Work in 30-minute increments.
Be still and silent.	Move your body.
Rest more!	Do more!

Chapter 18

How to Utilise Your Cycle

How did you go with your tracking? We are now getting into the part of the book where you can look at what you prefer to do in your seasonal weeks and utilise that knowledge!

After you are confident with what you prefer to do each week according to the seasons, you can move onto really utilising your cycle. A great way to use this section is to wait until you are going through each of the seasonal weeks and read the chapter that is relevant. That way you can journal what is happening for you and creatively come up with ideas on how you can utilise each week for yourself. Remember our cycles are all different, therefore, how you are feeling will be different. This is all about creating the self-awareness around how you work best!

Through each seasonal week we are going to look at the 10 areas on the sun we looked at in the Align section.

The 10 areas are:

- Physical environment

- Finances
- Work/career/business
- Relationships
- Romance
- Spirituality
- Personal growth/development/learning/education
- Health and wellness
- Fun and recreation
- Use of technology/social media/screen time

You may like to revisit this chapter to see what your goals were at the beginning of this book, or perhaps, do the activity again to see where you would like to focus your energy at this point in time. We will be allocating these 10 areas to your cycle to ensure that you are spending time on each of them. When we focus on these areas, we are more likely to shine brightly because all areas are being looked after.

Remember to be kind to yourself as you learn how you can utilise your energy cycle. There is no right way, and it does not have to be perfect. I review my cycle every month and still have seasonal weeks where I know I have not utilised them the best I could, but this is where my self-awareness kicks in and I ask myself, 'What do I need more of?' By looking at your cycle, you give yourself permission to repeat and trial.

A common question I am asked is, 'What happens when X and Y happen, and it doesn't fit in with your cycle?' Life does fit into your cycle because your cycle fits into your life. You may have a huge life event happen, so big that you really just want time to stop. If you have spent time using your masculine energy to set up structures for your feminine energy to flow, you can completely stop. Then you can allow your feminine energy to nurture and look after yourself, taking the time you need. We no longer have to be on the 'hamster wheel'. See your journey as a train ride in which you can choose when you are on the train and when you step off at the station.

When you know where your energy is going to be at different times of your cycle, you can set up supportive habits to help you be the best you can be at that certain time. My Autumn and Winter Weeks fall on Mothers' Day and Christmas Time. These are two times where I am expected to be at my highest energy and photo-ready at any moment. Well, I am not. So, I have learnt to really slow down in the Spring and Summer Weeks of these cycles, book my beauty appointments in advance and purchase the most beautiful clothes so then on the day I can feel my best (because these things make me feel good, you may have different things that make you feel good). I have birthdays that I often forget, are not prepared for or don't feel like attending because every year they fall in my Autumn and Winter Weeks. Once again, it has taken me time to recognise that there are reasons why going to an extended family event causes me a lot of anxiety and I feel more self-conscious than usual because every year my cycle has repeated itself. I even had my wedding during the transition between autumn and winter! If I knew what I know now, I would have easily booked it the complete opposite weekend in my cycle and in my spring and summer crossover!

Outside of our own seasonal weeks our environment experiences its own seasons. Up until this point, we may have viewed certain things only at a surface level. You may already schedule tasks/activities during the year because 'at a surface level' it is something that has been passed down from generations. Spring cleaning is an example of this. You may even have a farming background and organise your life according to the seasons because of the crops and animals. From a women's perspective, what if we were to look at the environment seasons at a deeper level? How can you utilise the environmental seasons? To continue with the theme of this book, I will be discussing the four seasons I have been working with. Please note my acknowledgement at the start of the book for the Traditional Custodians of the Land I live on and the Indigenous seasons. I would also like to recognise that the closer you live to the equator, the fewer seasons you experience.

Things to consider
SPRING • Clean, declutter and reorganise the house. • Prepare the back and front yard for warmer seasons. • Change over clothes for the warmer months. • Begin your plans to act on what you want to bring into your life. My major projects: • Go through each room in the house and reorganise and declutter. I write down a list of things I need to upgrade, update and renew. • Prepare for end of year and Christmas (Southern Hemisphere) • Finalise any business projects I am launching in Summer.

SUMMER

- Enjoy the goals you have set for yourself and achieved.
- Be active, get outside!
- Socialise and connect with others.
- Select the higher energy activities that you feel like you don't have time and energy for. There will be time to slow down in the months to come.

My major projects:
- Purchase the items on my upgrade list.
- Enjoy the Christmas period (Southern Hemisphere)
- Launch my business projects.

- Clean, declutter and reorganise the house. Imagine doing this twice a year rather than leaving it to one occasion.
- Go on family adventures and enjoy the weather cooling down.
- A time for reflection and celebration. Reflect on what is happening in your life. Celebrate what you have achieved.
- Prepare to start 'hibernating' or slowing down your life. Imagine harnessing this! If we allow ourselves to slow down, then we will feel like we have more time and energy.

My major projects:
- Brainstorm what I would like to create in my life and start to dream about what is possible.
- This is my health transformation period. After 2 masculine-dominated energy months, I revert to relying more on my feminine energy. So, looking after myself is important during this time. I focus on upleveling and transformation, which actually works well because the external world slows down.
- Make sure I catch up with friends and family so I can take some time out at home in winter.

WINTER

- Use this time to recharge. Use this time to actually stop and slow down. Give yourself permission to do so.
- Select the quieter tasks that you feel you do not have time for.
- Enjoy being at home and perhaps even do some additional jobs around the house.
- You may also like to use this time to take up study or learn something new.

My major projects:
- Enjoy being at home.
- Create beautiful memories with my kids at home.
- Experience and enjoy the wild weather! Yep, this is a big one for me. Why do we feel we have to stay out of the rain? When we can enjoy it, there is no bad weather, just bad clothing choices.

WORKING WITH THE MOON

I love recommending going outside at night to look up at the sky and track the moon. For so long I thought that the moon couldn't be seen and thought it was on the 'other side of the world', yep, even as an adult. I then started researching the moon cycles and realised that the moon was actually in the sky, it was just its position and the reflection (or lack of) and therefore called a new moon. You can use your menstrual cycle alongside the moon as discussed in Chapter 10. Working with the moon can be therapeutic and a powerful way to create more time and energy.

Imagine having a routine that worked with the moon where you could release things that are holding you back from creating the life you want to live. This is also a great time to get your hands on some crystals and have a little fun thinking you are magical, because you really are! This is also a great starting point if you don't have a menstrual cycle that you can track or you are pre-menopausal or menopausal. I particularly like following this ritual when I would like one specific thing to come into my life! Have some fun with this magic.

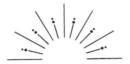

Suggested ritual or routine:

New Moon: The moon cannot be seen. Time to set some goals and intentions for what you would like this cycle.

Waxing Crescent: This is the beginning of new things. Time to start actioning your intentions.

First Quarter: Lots of magic around. Tick those things off your list.

Waxing Gibbous: Take a moment to reflect on the steps you have taken already. Are they going to support you in achieving your goal? Slow down for a couple of days to allow yourself to make the most of the energy that is about to come.

Full Moon: This is the midway point. You may feel extra emotional during this time. Be aware of what comes up for you. This also signals a time to slow down as you approach the end of the cycle.

Waning Gibbous: Time to start finishing your projects.

Last Quarter: A time for reassessing and reflecting. How did you go with achieving your goal or intention? Did the magic happen?

Waning Crescent: What can you learn from this cycle? What would you like from the next cycle?

Chapter 19

Utilise Your Winter Week

In my Winter Week I completely allow myself to indulge, be lazy and allow things to move slowly. This is the week I watch my television series that I used to wish I had time for. It is when I allow myself to sleep in and have a weekend with no plans. I reach for one of my books during this time and no longer feel guilt during the other weeks because I am not reading regularly. Something as simple as this makes such a huge difference. There were years where I didn't even read because I felt like I wasn't reading regularly so what was the point. Now I read at least 12 weeks out of the year. I schedule my writing tasks during this time and look ahead to see what is due in a couple of weeks. That way I am ahead of the schedule and often able to submit things earlier. I do want to mention here that it is important to not also hand work tasks in earlier. Sometimes doing things ahead of schedule results in you doing more things because you got it done earlier. We do not want to add to our list because our energy cycle will change, and we want to shift our focus to different types of tasks. So, hold onto the work you completed early and submit it when the due date arrives. That way you feel calm knowing that the job is done, and you will not increase your workload because you were being productive. This will also give you space to breathe and fit in other tasks.

Things to be aware of during your Winter Week:
- Your emotions tend to be close to the surface so an emotional response before logic is highly likely.
- Your body may be craving different types of comfort food, so it is probably best not to start new habits or healthy eating regimes during this week.
- Your energy will be like a yoyo and one minute you will feel strong and depleted the next. Make sure you schedule lots of down time between tasks and activities even if they do not seem too hard to do.
- When 'life happens' and your plan has to go out of the window, allow it to fly straight out, don't work against yourself and try to put another plan in place. Just select three major things you would like to achieve during the entire week and get them done. The rest can go on your list for the following week. Remember our energy cycle weeks do not always flow with the calendar week so you can re-adjust your timeframes to still suit.
- Really enjoy doing the slower paced tasks and the self-care activities that you 'wished' you had more time for.

THE 10 SUN AREAS:

Physical environment

This is the perfect time to appreciate your home. We often spend so much time working to create a home that we are often too busy to enjoy. Allow your Winter Week to be the week you enjoy your home!

Now take some time to brainstorm how you would like to enjoy your physical space during your Winter Week.

Finances

You may like to stay away from shopping during this time, that includes clothes and food. You may feel more impulsive and because you feel lower on energy, you may crave to 'fill yourself up'. Focus on 'filling yourself up' in a nourishing way.

Work/career/business

Note how you feel during this time when you are at work. Are you more emotional? Do you feel tired? Do you feel like socialising? How do you prefer to communicate, in person, on the phone, via email or message? What type of tasks do you prefer to do at work during this time? Are these jobs repeated regularly? Can you schedule them for approximately four weeks' time?

How do you prefer to communicate?
What jobs do you like to do during this time?
What jobs would you like to schedule in every Winter Week?

Relationships

You may find that you prefer to be an introvert during this time. Be okay with focusing on yourself and spending time alone. This is a great time to recharge so you have more to give in your other seasonal weeks. You may like to spend this week focusing on your relationship with yourself. When we want to see a change in our relationships, we first must focus on the change in ourselves. To change your external world, change your internal world first! So, you can brainstorm all the ways you would like others to treat you or what you want from other relationships and then treat yourself to these things during your Winter Week. A great example is having flowers delivered. Why wait for someone else to surprise yourself with flowers when you can organise it yourself.

What would you like more of in other relationships?
How you can show yourself these things?

Romance

What does romance mean to you? This is taking your relationships one step further and looking at what love means to you. Once again, start with yourself and then look outwards at others. How are you showing love? How are you receiving love? This is not the best time to have the conversation with others. The majority of clients I work with will explain that it is during their Winter Week where they are more than likely to have a fight with their partners. Use your Winter Week to reflect and think about your romantic situation and simply make note of how you would like it to look. What would you like more of? What would you like less of? Use this as a time to learn about love rather than enforce it. We all receive and feel love in different ways, you may like to do an online quiz on your love language and potentially find out your partner's and children's. Your Winter Week is a great time to really fill your love cup up!

List some ways for you to feel the love:

❤	❤
❤	❤
❤	❤
❤	❤
❤	❤

Spirituality

During your Winter Week you will intuitively feel more connected. If you like all things spiritual but aren't sure where to start or find you are too busy to dive in deep and enjoy, this is the perfect week to do so. If you would like to start a regular spiritual practise, start this week (unlike healthy lifestyle changes). Look at the both the mental and physical spiritual tools you have and take some time to play, connect and listen.

Personal growth/development/learning/education

Your Winter Week is a fantastic week for you to dive into that personal development book you have been wanting to read. Start or continue the online course you purchased. Listen to the podcasts in your library. You may have a selection of resources or studies that you would like to continue but seem to be relegated to the bottom of the list when all the other things take over. Because of this, it's a really good idea to have a pile, file or folder that houses all your courses, books and podcasts. That way, when you hit your Winter Week, you can just pull out the folder and dive into something that interests you. You may even like to schedule these things in advance so you know what you will be learning during this time. If you are still at school, college or university, your Winter Week is great for writing notes, reading and doing all the preparation for exams and assignments.

Health and wellness

Discipline will be hard during this time. Making radical lifestyle changes will also be difficult. You can still dream and do your research. During this week, you may like to brainstorm what type of healthy lifestyle you want. What would you like to do more of? What would you like to do less of? This is a time where you may be feeling more inclined to research and learn, collect new recipes or look for inspiration. Winter is all about preparing for Spring, so use this time to do your research, planning and preparation so you can launch into your Spring Week well-informed and ready to go!

Know that you will prefer to eat heavier meals during this time, so make sure you are stocked up on healthier choices that are still going to hit the 'cravings' on the head. You may also not feel like exercising so opt to do slower pace exercise and know that exercise can often reduce headaches and cramps.

Fun and recreation

You can still have fun and participate in recreation during this time. It is just a matter of what types of activities you feel like doing. Fun activities may be watching television, reading a book or doing some other activity at home. Just list the ways you would like to have fun in your Winter Week and then refer to them. If you do this for each seasonal week, you will be able to allocate all the things you find enjoyable across the week without feeling like you don't have enough time or motivation.

Use of technology/social media/screen time

You will feel drawn to use more technology and have screen time. Utilise this time. Allow yourself to catch up on the series or movies you have been wanting to watch, and sit there without your phone in your hand, and enjoy watching them. Don't feel guilty for not doing things—that time will come. Be aware when you are on social media, if you find yourself scrolling and comparing, decide to edit your profile and go through your own feed. Use technology with intention.

Chapter 20

Utilise Your Spring Week

In my Spring Week I totally overload my to-do list, but I have a specific focus. It may be something like getting the house cleaned and organised or getting my business documents up to date, then breaking down the bigger tasks into smaller ones so I can start allocating them to specific days of the week. Since I tend to be up for socialising and catching up with friends at the end of the week, I schedule to call them or arrange a catch up during that time. I don't fall into the habit of booking the whole week out with social arrangements anymore because I actually want time in my office to get things done.

The other thing I do is wake up earlier and allow myself plenty of time to get to any appointments. Because I am in a super productive mood, I will not only do one task at a time, but I will also start lots of tasks because I feel in flow. Sometimes this means I finish and hang a load of washing when I am supposed to have left 15 minutes ago. My Spring Week is when I feel the best about my body, and I have the exercise and strength to make healthy choices. It is a great time to start a new health regime or habit and try on new clothes. I once mentioned this to a client at one of my workshops and she scheduled a shopping spree during her Spring Week. She reached out to thank me because now all month she feels fabulous because the clothes she chose during that time were fun and colourful. How many items are in your wardrobe that are black or don't fit properly? I wonder what week of your cycle you went shopping…

Things to be aware of during your Spring Week:

- Overcommitting and trying to do too much. This does take some time to master but every month you will work towards finding the right balance.
- You may not want to spend time with the kids because you want to be productive. I like to reach into my 'mum' file and have a couple of activities with the kids planned for the week.
- You feel good and look good—own that confidence!
- Really zone into what you want to achieve during this cycle. You can plan ahead knowing that you will have 12 Spring Weeks in a year… so what are 12 major tasks you would like to achieve?
- Sometimes you will feel your Spring Week will be 'low' on energy. It is actually not low, instead, your spring energy wants to flow somewhere else. Your brain might want it on different tasks, but your body will want it to go somewhere else. Allow yourself to stop and focus on where it wants to go, you will be pleasantly surprised.

THE 10 SUN AREAS:

Physical environment

This is a great time to reorganise and declutter. If you have any major projects you want to get done in this time, these are the weeks to schedule them. Think of 10 to 12 house projects you want done in a year and schedule them to start in these weeks.

You might like to use my room planner as you work your way through the house to decide what you would like to achieve.

ROOM PLANNER

Room:

Things to Do		Things to Upgrade	
Things to Sell	Things to Donate		Things to Buy

Finances

Allocate time to review your finances and set goals. This is a great time to deal with paperwork and filing. You may like to make finances one of your above 'home projects'. Create systems and structures (great for harnessing the masculine energy in this seasonal week) so you know where your finances are at.

You may like to take some time reflecting on your finances:

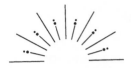

How do you feel about money?
What do you need to organise when it comes to your money?
What are your financial goals and how are you going to
achieve them?

Work/career/business

Be prepared to also get things done at work. Now is the time to have a prioritised to-do list. You may like to refer to Chapter 25 where I go through some organisational structures.

Relationships

It is not like you won't care about your relationships in this time—you will enjoy seeing people—it's just that you are in more of a 'doing' energy rather than a 'taking up time' energy. This is a great time to invite people to catch up next week.

Romance

As a result of harnessing a lot of masculine energy in this time, romance is a great opportunity to offset that energy by bringing more feminine energy to the balance. Romance is a great area to direct this energy because you will be feeling great and looking really good! Supercharge your feminine energy by tapping into all things beauty, indulgence, sexy and fun in the romance department! Not to mention, great stress relief and a quick way to bring you back into your body when you are getting lots of things done and spending a lot of time in your head during the day.

Spirituality

It would be an ideal situation to focus on your spiritual practices to keep your balance in check. This may be the time where you just do a few key practices to remind you of the importance of being grounded and not overdoing it.

You can write 3 key spiritual practices you would like to do on a daily basis during your Spring Week.

Personal growth/development/learning/education

It is okay to put your learning at the bottom of the priority list in this week. It is actually a week where you use what you have learnt and put it into action.

Health and wellness

Ensure you do not get so busy that you forget or don't prioritise your health and wellness goals. You will naturally feel stronger and fitter, plus you will feel better in your clothes and not have cravings for different foods. If you find yourself reaching for foods you prefer not to eat, this may be a good sign that you are overworking your Spring Week energy and the best choice would be to slow down and take a break. If you want to start a new health regime, this is the week to do it because you will be disciplined, your hormones will be as evenly balanced as possible and your mindset will be more on the positive, 'can-do' side, which will get you off to a good start!

Fun and recreation

You will have the energy to have fun but perhaps will opt to use the time to work more. It is up to you really and where your priorities are. You may like to spend this week organising all the fun things you can do next week.

Use of technology/social media/screen time

Firstly, who has time to watch television when you are feeling so productive!

Secondly, if you are using your laptop or phone a lot, please get some good blue light glasses.

Thirdly, selfie time! Though only if you want to. This is the time where you will probably be doing 'cool' things where you want to share them on social media. You will also be feeling good about yourself so more likely to post photos of yourself. Once again, be aware of your intention. You may be in your highest energy cycle week but someone who is looking on their social media feed where you pop up may be in their lowest. Now I don't want this to sound like I am telling you not to post on social media at all, rather be aware and have an intention. If you are happier to post on social media in this time, would you be happy posting in your Autumn Week too? Social media has a lot to answer for when it comes to mental health. So, when you go to post all those amazing photos and show how fantastic your life is… I am totally up for that and cheering you on because you should take a moment to celebrate how wonderful your life is. Just take a moment to recognise that there may be times you can post the opposite feeling (please also be aware of what you are posting at all times, the good, the bad and the ugly) or perhaps during your Autumn Week you can go and comment positive things on those photos that are triggering you, so you balance it all out.

*Take a moment now to create an intention
with your use of social media*

My intention with social media is to:
During my Spring Week I will:
During my Summer Week I will:
During my Winter Week I will:
During my Autumn Week I will:

Chapter 21

Utilise Your Summer Week

During my Summer Week I can start to feel my energy slow down. I am still high on energy, but my energy is directed more to socialising and getting out and about. I no longer feel like actioning things in my office, and I prefer to complete smaller tasks rather than get into larger ones. This is the week where I like going to appointments and doing the tasks that get me out of the house. I am also very happy to catch up with friends and feel like I can communicate effectively. I love to play and have fun during this week. It is a good week for me to dance around more and be in my feminine energy. It feels really good to turn up the feminine energy during this week after being so productive in my masculine week. I like to think of my Spring Week as my masculine energy-dominated week and my Summer Week as my feminine energy-dominated week, this brings me more into my ideal balance.

Things to be aware of during your summer week:

- It is best to finish off the projects you started in the spring week and transfer any that are not important to the following week.
- Socialising and talking with friends and family will come naturally.
- It is a really good week for promoting your best version of yourself.
- You will naturally feel more confident and fearless.
- This is the week to really have fun! Go all out! You might want to do things to remind you that you are still you!

THE 10 SUN AREAS:

Physical environment

Time to enjoy being outdoors rather than spending time organising your house. If you still have rooms and piles to sort out, please be okay with leaving them there until your next Spring Week.

Finances

You will be more likely to want to spend money during this time. Have a look at the budget you created last seasonal week and ensure you have a plan so you can enjoy your money without spending it all.

Work/career/business

Time to schedule fewer tasks this week and look at more tasks that require the communication side. This is a great week to book meetings, phone/zoom calls and attend networking events. If you have to promote or share what you are doing, schedule it for this week.

Relationships

Bring on all the socialising! Schedule it all for this week (and at the end of the Spring Week). Have fun!

Romance

Keep riding the romance train! This is a great time to have conversations that you have been wanting to have. Especially because you have been previously focused on connection and now the fun side. I recommend having these conversations now so when you feel more emotional over the next two weeks, they are less likely to come out, plus you are really strong with communication at this point of your cycle.

Take a moment to brainstorm some
ideas about the conversations you
would like to have.

You may also like to venture out to asking what your partner would like more from you and what they want in their life so you can ensure that you are growing together rather than apart.

Spirituality

Once again, you might like to refer to those three main spiritual practices you would like to continue this week.

Personal growth/development/learning/education

What would you like to learn about next? You will be coming into a cycle where you gravitate to internal tasks and learning is a great time for those two energy cycle weeks.

Take some time to write down the
current things you are learning about and
what you would like to learn about:

What are you currently learning?
What courses have you paid for that you have not
had time to complete?
What would you like to learn about?
How are you going to access that learning?
Who would you like to work with?

Health and wellness

This is a great time to establish what type of healthy lifestyle you would like to have. You have had a couple of weeks where you have felt very successful when it comes to food and exercise choices. Now is to find the balance you are seeking. When you are looking at yourself holistically, what would you like to do to nourish your mind, body and soul?

Fun and recreation

Time to remember that you are a person living your own life! You know those moments when you are fully present and having a great time and you remind yourself that you are living? I feel this every time I am snorkelling or on a carnival ride—it must have something to do with the mix of adrenaline and stepping outside my comfort zone. What would your life be like if you incorporated more fun like this on a regular basis? This is one of the reasons that I love to encourage the #swingchallenge in the Lead and Inspire Community. Every time you see a swing, get on it and have some fun! Please send photos to me, tag me on social media @jessicaterlick and post in our Facebook groups because I truly believe that this will encourage more women to have fun!

Journaling 🦋 prompts

- Take a moment to walk down memory lane and write down all the things you enjoyed and had fun doing when you were a kid.
- Now take a moment to write down all the things you enjoyed at a teenager.
- Now take a moment to write down all the things you enjoyed or are enjoying now as an adult
- What would you like to try?
- What would be fun for you?

Use of technology/social media/screen time

You will find your Summer Week very similar to your Spring Week in most of the areas above. Your use of technology, social media and screen time will also be very similar to your Spring Week. Towards the end of your Summer Week, you may start to find yourself wanting time to watch television and 'chill out', just know that that time is coming.

Chapter 22

Utilise Your Autumn Week

Mastering how to utilise my Autumn Week is still a challenge for me. As I write this book, I am finding that I am actually reducing my Autumn Week to only 4 days and I am yet to know if this is positive or negative. I feel that I am doing this because I completely stop as soon as I feel my energy switch from summer energy to autumn energy. This allows my body to get the rest it needs in preparation for releasing in my Winter Week. Whilst I rest, I review and celebrate, I honour and I show gratitude. It is a beautiful celebration of the month that has been and the magic and power I was able to use. So, I utilise this phase by not doing much at all and doing the things that I wished I had more time for like watching television, going to beauty appointments and having a really small to-do list.

Things to be aware of during your Autumn Week:
- Panic and anxiety can set in if you have not given

yourself permission to go slow down this week.

- Social media is more likely to trigger negative emotions and put you in a position where you start to compare yourself to others. It is at this point that I like to look at my own social media and work instead to reflect and review. I examine what I would like to change while acknowledging the good things I am doing too.
- It is a good time to leave other people reviews, send testimonials, thank people and show random acts of kindness.
- You may like to use this week to clear out emails and messages.
- It is okay if you are not feeling the best about yourself. Be kind, gentle and loving towards yourself.

THE 10 SUN AREAS:
Physical environment

During your Autumn Week you may like to spend some time doing any last-minute organisation around your home and car. You might like to get your car washed or detailed. This is a great week to pay for services so if you would like to organise a monthly cleaning or gardening service, your Autumn Week would be a good time to do this. The main thing with your physical environment is to ensure that all your systems and structures are in place so your household can run by itself for a couple of weeks.

You might like to:
- Set up a food delivery service or get your food

shopping delivered.
- Bulk-cook meals and do some forward planning for lunchtime snacks.
- Ensure your washing is up to date and the house has had a good clean.

Finances

Avoid online shopping and buying things on impulse. As your energy drops you may feel like boosting yourself by purchasing items. Make sure you are buying with the right intention. I have had members opt to make their Autumn Week their savings week.

Work/career/business

Try to finish tasks and projects you have started. Switch to more of a learning and listening mode rather than doing. Look for ways to show appreciation to others and acknowledge the work others are doing. Rather than looking at what others are achieving, take a moment to acknowledge and celebrate what you have achieved and completed this month. During this week you may spell words incorrectly when you otherwise know to spell them and jumble your words when you speak.

You might like to:
- Reduce your to-do list.
- Send thank you cards or messages to others.
- Take a break from your work if it is possible.

Relationships

Be aware that you may be more emotional than usual. This is the week where find things upset you more than normal. Just be in the moment when you are with others. If things upset you, take time to process what it means to you, see it from the other person's point of view and decide whether it needs to be addressed right now or in a seasonal week where you will be able to communicate more effectively. You may like to retreat to doing more independent activities and say no to any social invites.

<u>Romance</u>

You may start to feel the need to pull away and be by yourself. This can be confusing to others, especially if you have been 'on' for the last two weeks. Create conversation around what is happening for you at this time of your cycle and how it makes you feel. Encourage other gestures such as cuddling and holding hands to create connection still. When we become busy, these gestures are often forgotten but can make such a difference to a relationship.

<u>Spirituality</u>

You will feel closer to your intuition at this time. Take a moment to really connect. Schedule in quiet time, journaling and time outside.

<u>Personal growth/development/learning/education</u>

As you may feel like doing independent activities this is the week to open up what you want to learn. So, schedule the courses you want to work on or the study you want to (or have to) complete in this week. Put a podcast on when you are doing a task you prefer not to do.

Health and wellness

Be kind and gentle but still move during this time. Schedule lower impact movement. You may like to allow yourself to eat the foods you opt not to for the majority of the week and really enjoy them rather than feeling guilty. This area of the sun is really important in supporting you to switch over to more of a feminine energy structure as you have been operating a lot from your masculine energy over the last couple of weeks. Really indulge in a lot of self-care activities that boost your health and wellness.

Fun and recreation

You will still want to have fun, just a different type of fun. Schedule the activities that you want to do more of but are slower pace—quieter, more nurturing and nourishing.

Use of technology/social media/screen time

Try to avoid anything that is going to make you feel inadequate. Use this time to detox from technology or go through all your inboxes and messages and delete what isn't necessary. Sort out your virtual space instead of going down the 'rabbit hole'.

Chapter 23

Guilt, Judgement and Comparison

Let's take a moment to talk about guilt. I didn't realise how much time I spent feeling guilt as a woman and even a young girl. When I was a young girl, I experienced guilt for being too loud, not being consistently nice to everyone, not doing what everyone wanted me to do, not looking a certain way, then for achieving too much, doing too much and spending time on my studies rather than going out with my boyfriend and friends. At the time, I didn't realise that this was guilt. I thought I was just feeling bad about myself. Then when I was at university, I experienced guilt when it came to what I ate and how I looked; I felt guilty because I didn't know all the answers, but everyone thought I did because I came across confident; I even felt guilty because I didn't like the music that my peers liked. Now that I reflect on this guilt, I believe that I experienced it because I did not know or understand who I truly was, and I felt guilty about that. I was not speaking or acting my truth, I was trying to be what others wanted me to be and to please others by doing what I thought they wanted me to do.

Completely unaware of this growing guilt, I experienced it more when I became a teacher. I felt guilty for not feeling like I met the needs of every single student, I felt guilty because I felt like I wasn't doing enough and then I felt guilty for feeling guilty rather than just getting it all done. This completely exhausted me. Then I would feel guilty for sitting on the couch after work, unable to move and then finally work up enough strength to cook myself some dinner. Meanwhile I had set myself a huge to-do list to complete at home in preparation for the next day. I felt guilty for not covering everything I had planned to do or not put in place every good idea that I saw. As a result, I modified and refined what I was doing. I looked at what was working and what wasn't, and I started to make changes. But these were all externally related. I didn't look within or connect with who I was, I pushed harder to achieve what I believed I needed to do in order to please those around me. No surprises where that left me, and I am sure you can relate, that first job that you completely set out to prove yourself, how did you end up after it, or if you are going through it now, how are you really feeling.

I truly felt the real guilt when I became a mum. Mum guilt is certainly a thing. Especially when you are driven to do the best in every role you have. I felt guilty for not being the teacher that I once was because I was working part-time, then I felt guilty because I went to work a couple of days a week and enjoyed it. Eventually I felt guilty because I didn't feel like I was giving anything or anyone 100 per cent. My breaking point, the point in which I decided to get off the guilt train, was when my emotional responses were no longer aligned with the reaction to certain events. I have always been known for crying. Crying is often my response to being angry, and then I get angry for crying, and then cry more. I have now decided to embrace this; I am an emotionally strong and passionate woman. It was a key moment where I felt like no matter what I was doing, no one was getting the best of me, not even myself. I was burnt out and felt so guilty for not being the person I truly wanted to be.

I decided to use my journal to start writing down who I really wanted to be. I didn't look for other examples, I didn't think about what others wanted me to be, I decided who I wanted to be by looking within and considering what felt right to me. I started with how I wanted to feel and then connected it to what made me feel this way. Then I looked at what I was required to do at this certain stage of my life or season of my life and that was work part time whilst my children were young. I then accepted where I was and the resources I had at the time. I turned my attention to being grateful for what I had and the opportunities I created. With the aspects of my life that I was not happy with, I looked at ways to slowly change them. Interestingly enough, the things that I felt guilty about were the things that I was not happy with.

Now, for me, I felt like most of my guilt now was connected to home and my children. I was guilty about not keeping the house the way I wanted, I was guilty that I wasn't playing with the children enough, I was guilty about the food I ate, I felt guilty about how much time I spent on my business, and I was guilty about how I felt tired and exhausted all the time.

So, I started to plan my home and family focuses around my seasonal weeks. I tuned into my cycle, and I was able to work out the weeks that I did feel like playing with the children versus the week I preferred them to play together or independently. I soon realised that it was my Summer and Autumn Weeks that I felt most inclined to play the games they wanted and then the Spring and Winter Weeks where I preferred to do the things I planned and have them occupy themselves. This was absolutely perfect because I no longer felt guilty. I knew that as a result of my energy cycle I did not feel like playing with my children the way I believed I should, and it wasn't because I was being lazy, inconsistent or a bad mum.

My Spring Week is all about house organisation because as you might have guessed, that is the week where I actually feel like 'spring cleaning'. Have you ever noticed that week where you are busy doing a task you then open a cupboard or a drawer or fridge and suddenly just decide to pull everything out and reorganise it? Chances are you didn't expect to do it, you certainly didn't plan it, and there is a possibility you did it because you may be running late for something else, but you felt oh so good after doing it—a real sense of achievement. This is a true indicator of being in your Spring Week. So, when it came to decluttering and reorganising the house, I only scheduled to do one room every Spring Week. So yes, it took me a whole year, but you know the beauty with decluttering? It keeps your space organised more often. If my Spring Week landed in the school holidays, I would do the whole house in that week just as a reset. As a result, for the other weeks of the year I no longer felt drained by the thought of having a messy house and a spare bedroom or cupboard that I really needed to sort out.

I was able to allocate everything I felt guilty about to one week or more weeks to my energy cycle. Once these things had time allocated to them, I was focused and in the present moment doing the tasks. Soon enough the feeling of consistency amplified because I know I was doing something rather than wishing I could or feeling guilty that I wasn't.

We are told that we need to be consistent in order to be successful. How about we be flexible with our consistency and allow it to roll with our energy cycle? I would like you to refer to it as flexible consistency.

Where are you currently feeling guilty in life? Take a moment to write down in your journal all the things you feel guilty about. Forgive yourself. Then look at ways you can incorporate more of these things into life by looking at your seasonal weeks.

Guilt can be a biproduct of judgement. We have no reason to feel guilty if we have no judgements. When we judge, we highlight something inside of us that wants to be seen. Judgement can also come from comparing yourself and your journey to others. Guilt, judgement and comparison are all time and energy suckers! As women, we are encouraged to judge, compare and feel guilty. All three things keep us small, encourage us to stay in our comfort zone and stay quiet by keeping us in a state of anxiousness, burnout and overwhelm. I know, big call, right? What if we could see that every time we judge ourselves or someone else we are keeping ourselves small? What if we could see that every time we compare, we are setting women up to work *against* each other rather than *with* each other. What if we could see that when we experience guilt, we are giving our energy away to thoughts that do not serve us.

I judge and compare more during my Autumn and Winter Weeks. It is like my brain is purposely trying to find things that I feel like I am not good at or things I need to improve. But I am in control of what my brain searches for. Somewhere along my timeline I have told my brain what I want to be, do or have, while passing judgement and comparing this to others. Now when I find myself judging and comparing, I look at it as an opportunity to ask myself, 'Is this something I really want in my life?' And if it is, I can write down how I can make it happen rather than allow that energy to stay and make me feel bad about myself (and then reach for the sweet treats). If it is not something I actually want, then I interrupt my thinking to show my brain that yes, that looks great (even take a moment to let that person know) and then look for other things that I actually want in my life.

You know that saying 'The grass is not always greener on the other side'? I prefer the upgraded version of it: 'The grass is greener where you water it'. This might mean more to me as my husband runs an elite lawn service and our lawn is incredibly green, but this is all a constant reminder that my grass is green because I take the time to water it (not my actual lawn, that is Ben's love). So, when I spiral into judging and comparing, I know that there is something I need to water inside of me, just like when I use my rain water tank metaphor in the Align section—see how wonderfully those metaphors marry up!

I spent a lot of time in my teenage years judging, comparing and even tearing others down. I have no excuses for it, and I am deeply apologetic for doing it. But I now know why I did it. I didn't have a deep understanding of my energy cycle—I actually had no understanding at all. So, when I was feeling 'low' I was attracted to making others around me feel low. What if, as women, when we feel low, we choose to make others feel 'high'? Imagine that transfer of energy! Can we agree on raising, boosting and totally elevating each other by knowing our very own feminine energy cycle as our very own superpower? How lucky are we to know that we can harness our own energy and use it to create the life we truly want? If we reduce the feeling of guilt, recognise that judgment and comparison are ways of establishing what we really want in life, and that we can choose to raise others, then magic will definitely happen!

Chapter 24

Recreating What Time Means

I have always loved the traditional calendar and timetable. Something about the structure makes me feel safe. Over the last couple of years and particularly once I started focusing on my natural feminine energy cycle, I have started to see the traditional forms of time as restrictive, counterproductive and very supportive of the masculine energy cycle.

Knowing that this book will not change how we schedule our calendars, clocks and traditional work hours, I would prefer to invite you to look at time differently. One of the number one problems my coaching clients have when they come to me is that they feel like they don't have enough time. What if we looked at time differently? What if we officially started our week on a different day? For example, the day our cycle changes. You may go to work on a Monday and finish on a Friday, but your perspective of time can stretch and look at your week as Thursday to Wednesday.

When I returned to work after having my children, I officially started my week on a Sunday. You will still find some calendars starting on a Sunday. For me, starting on a Sunday made sense because it was the one day of the week where I was completely in control of what I did on the day. I could start my day slowly, spend it with my loved ones and choose the activities I felt like doing. What a fantastic way to start my week! I often share my Sunday afternoon routine with my Lead and Inspire Community. I begin with meal prepping and getting dinner done, writing out my weekly check-in and to-do list, then taking the family out for a walk or play afterwards to break the cycle of worrying about what I need to do for the rest of the week Then on Monday when I went to work, I would still feel content (because I filled my cup the day before) about the week and know that my week was set up for success because each task was allocated for each day. I must say though, I do love Mondays, anyway! I love Mondays because I have the rest of the week to look forward to and plenty of time to get things completed!

If you were to align your weeks to your cycle, then you may not actually start your week on a Monday. Knowing this, you can schedule different tasks according to your natural energy cycle for example, rather than cleaning your house at the start of the week when you are in winter, plan it for at the end when that spring energy comes into play!

As my cycle changes, I look at the month ahead differently. I set intentions according to my menstrual cycle rather than looking at what I want to achieve in the month. Let's take it one step further. What if we felt like our New Year was actually in March? That the festive period was a way of celebrating the end of the year and then we gave ourselves the first couple of months to settle into the flow what the year will be like and what we wanted to achieve.

What if we took it another step further and looked at the seasons? When I explain this, I will refer to the southern hemisphere since I live in Australia, but please flip the seasons if you live in the northern hemisphere. I have just gone through how our menstrual cycles go through the seasons and how we feel according to what we do in the actual seasons. Now what if we were to learn from our menstrual cycle and treat the actual seasons with the wisdom we have learnt? For example, summer is a time to celebrate, socialise and connect. Summer is about reaping the rewards. What if we focused on doing these things in the months of summer? Then autumn, a time to finish off, reflect and release what is no longer serving you. It is all about slowing down and once again celebrating what you have achieved in the busier months (spring and summer). Whereas winter is a time to hibernate, recalibrate and do the inner work. Take this time to reflect on who you are and how your year is going. Then spring is the time to act on new ideas (that were envisioned during winter), get things done and use the energy your conserved during winter.

Back in Chapter 17 you would remember I spoke about how time takes up the space you give it and to organise 'time-tasks' which are basically sub-tasks of the task. Remember to allocate these sub tasks to the seasonal week in which you will feel more in flow to complete them. Knowing that a task will take as long as the time you give it can be used to your advantage. You may decide to leave a task closer to when it is due and focus on what is the highest priority right now. You may experience less anxiety or even guilt when you have allocated each time-task to your seasonal week, and you know that when this task is due you will spend the last hours polishing it and making sure it is of the best quality. Imagine having something completed with the feeling of satisfaction and success.

During my Setting Your Year Up For Success workshop I ask participants to write down what is currently occupying their spaces. There is something about the jobs we have at home that we often put off because we do not feel like we have enough time. You do have the time. It is just that the task is not a high priority. If you allocate a motivator to the task, then you are more likely to place priority on the task. If you have a task you want to complete at home, set a due date for yourself. You may even like to host a catch up with family and friends to have this task completed. Work your way backwards and allocate the subtasks according to your seasonal weeks. With the motivation of the event and knowing that the house will be organised before then, you will be in a situation where you feel success. Some things to consider here include making sure your event is in your Spring Week and maybe even book a cleaner the week before and after the event to really celebrate your achievement!

There are so many different ways that you can create more time and have the energy to make things happen. You may like to follow this simple flow chart to remind yourself.

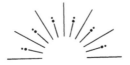

Select your intention. What is it that you
want to get done?

Set yourself a due date and have some sort
of motivating factor at the end.

Break the task into smaller time-tasks.

Allocate the time-tasks to your seasonal week.
Make sure you are utilising your energy cycle.

Just focus on the one task at a time.

Enjoy going through each time-task with ease,
flow and enjoyment.

Enjoy that celebration when you get to
the end of the task.

Chapter 25
Organisational Systems

When we utilise our masculine energy structures, our feminine energy is supported and will flow with ease. I love having a repertoire of organisational skills that I can rely on. You will notice that you have your own set of organisational structures. Recognise and celebrate this! Only you can decide for yourself what you need in order to feel organised. Each of us are different with different lives to run.

Journaling prompts

- Think of what structures you use.
- Think of what stationery you use.
- Think of what technology you use.
- Think about your support network.

Now think if any of this change depending on what seasonal week you are in. I don't know about you, but I own a lot of stationery! I love stationery so much that I even designed my own. I have stationery that I use every week to be organised and then stationery that I only use in different weeks. For example, I have a small to-do list pad that I use in my Winter Week because I feel overwhelmed when I look at my weekly planner and to-do book, that overwhelm soon becomes frustration because I just want to start actioning my to-do list but yet my energy cycle is still in rest and recharge mode. So, by having a small to-do list I am still productive without feeling overwhelmed or feel like I have too much to do.

I would like to share with you 4 organisational systems that absolutely work a treat for me through each stage of my energy cycle. I do have a range of stationery that I use behind the scenes as part of my masculine structures. You can check these out on my website www.jessicaterlick.com.au

SPRING: THE PRIORITISED TO-DO LIST!

This is my go-to prioritised list for when I feel overwhelmed. You do not always need this resource in order to set it out (you can if you like). That is the beauty of the system.

As you will see, my table has 5 sections.

QABCD

What does the QABCD System stand for?

- Q stands for Quick. It is here where you write all the quick activities you need to complete. These activities should not take any longer than 10 minutes.

- A is for the list of tasks with the highest priority. These are the tasks that need to be done as soon as possible.
- B is for the tasks that are a high priority but are due a bit later on in the week.
- C is for the tasks that you want to write down, so you don't forget them. They are not a high priority, but they will be if you don't get them done.
- D is for.... 'Don't even worry about it!'. If you must write something down in this list then follow the Do, Delete, Delegate or Delay method.
- Once your list is organised, take some time to appreciate what you have created. Then complete 1 or 2 items off your Q list to get your motivation pumping and then start tackling your A list! You've got this!

Q(UICK)	A	B	C	D

SUMMER: SIMPLE TO-DO LIST

During my Summer Week I like to be able to simplify everything and have it with me each day so I can see what I need to do, who I need to contact, what I need to organise and what I have to pay/buy.

TO DO - Day:	To Contact
	To Organise
	To Pay or Buy

AUTUMN: THE 4 DS

This is a great system that works really quickly. As you enter your Autumn Week it is a good idea to reduce your to-do list further and only retain what is high priority. To do this, you simply transfer what is on all your lists to this quadrant.

Do: What is high priority and still needs to be done?

Delegate: What can you get someone else to do for you? Who on your support team can help you?

Delete (my favourite): What can you delete? What can you drop that will release energy back to you? Remember these things are occupying your spaces and therefore using energy, even if you are not thinking about them all the time. So, release it! Drop it! Delete it!

Delay: What would you still like to complete but know that you are not in the right energy cycle for? What will be a high priority soon? These items can then be transferred to the Spring: Prioritised to-do list.

Do	Delegate
Delete	Delay

WINTER: THE 'WHAT I FEEL LIKE DOING' LIST

This is a nice simple list where you can select what you would like to do, depending on how you are feeling. You can adjust the titles to suit the areas you would like to focus on.

For me my areas are:

- Home and kids
- Self-care
- Work tasks
- Fun

So, my list will look something like this.

What I Feel Like Doing List			
Work Tasks	**Self-Care**	**Home**	**Kids**
Fun	**Learning for the Week**	**Select a thing:**	
		Podcast	
		Read	
		TV	
		Create	
		Outside	

Part 4

Share Your Shine

Chapter 26

Personal Safety vs. Feeling Safe

I spent 2017 focusing on my own health and raising my two babies. I joined an inspirational mum workout group, and it completely opened my eyes to looking after myself and learning about myself again. One day I heard a quote that changed everything: 'A ship is not built to stay in the harbour'.

This may not resonate with you the same way it resonated with me. But that is the thing, when you are ready to hear the message or learn the lesson from a teacher, both the message or the teacher will present themselves. I have always felt like I can do bigger things. I have always felt like there was a bigger purpose. We all have a purpose. And they are all big to us. Our purpose is not to be compared to anyone else's. When I took more time to think about what the ship staying in the harbour meant to me, I soon started thinking about the damage the ship could potentially incur by staying tied up. How one day the ship would be brand new and as time passed the ship would age yet never be fully utilised! If the ship was to be utilised, it would have travelled, it would have left that harbour to visit other harbours, it would have experienced adventures, learned, listened, and loved! And I wanted to do all these things too!

At this point in time, it was the right moment for me start taking the next step to share my shine! I had spent time creating a supportive toolkit of strategies and had a wealth of knowledge to share. The only thing stopping me was the feeling of safety. There is a difference between feeling safe and needing to be safe. When we step outside our doors, we certainly want to feel personal safety, so we do not hurt ourselves or be hurt by others. But when we try to keep ourselves safe inside our mind, we can be damaging ourselves.

'Growth and comfort do not coexist'. (Ginni Rometty)

Our brains are structured to keep us safe. Back when humans were not at the top of the food chain, our list of predators was quite longer than the list we have today. However, that function still exists, and we are triggered regularly and reminded to keep safe. This is to keep us in our comfort zone. I love my comfort zone. I love spending some time there. But I also know what happens when I stay in my comfort zone for too long. I start to sabotage myself and turn on my autopilot switch! This is when I stop living in the present moment. This is when I go to bed at night and wonder where the day has gone. This is when Friday rolls around again and I wonder where has the week, the month, the year has gone.

Yeah, no thank you.

So, it is important for me to regularly step outside of my comfort zone. I choose what I want to achieve and only did one thing at a time to avoid feeling overwhelmed or at risk of burnout. If I am tackling something at school, working on a project or getting a major task done, I will make sure that I am not trying to do a massive project for my business. If I have a week coming up that is busier than usual, I make sure that I only select three major focuses for the week and reduce the number of activities that I plan to do.

When a project requires me to step outside of my comfort zone, it is hard work! First comes the flooding of emotions and negative self-talk: *this is too hard, who do you think you are, you are not going to be able to do this, why are you doing this again?*

The more I am stepping outside my comfort zone, the louder the chatter, the bigger the emotions and the more I have the potential to snap. I start to think that I do not have enough time, that I am not good enough and I don't have enough energy. The key word here is *enough*. And when I start to feel this way, I go back to the beginning (even to the beginning of this book), and I give myself permission to stop. I stop. I select what strategies will be most supportive to me. I look at the cycle stage I am in. I think about what needs to be done and look for when I can utilise my energy cycle best with what I want to achieve. The 'why'… so I can share my shine!

STEPPING OUTSIDE YOUR COMFORT ZONE

Stepping outside your comfort zone and feeling comfortable with change are two ways you can support your natural energy cycle. If you become comfortable with feeling uncomfortable, growth will occur. One of our core abilities is the ability to keep us safe. It is a primal need that has wired our brains to create a feeling of safety. Did you know that our body's response to both fear and excitement is the same? It is our brain that decides which category this falls into. So, our brain creates a variety of patterns, structures and beliefs that create this 'comfort zone'. Anything that is not 'normal' or within the parameters of the comfort zone, an alarm is raised, and a body's response is released. If you act on it straight away, you are more than likely to retreat back into your comfort zone. If you choose to be curious and observe what has been triggered, then you can be empowered with the next choice you make. Proceed, detour or retreat.

I like to use a simple diagram of how your comfort zone looks:

 Hi comfort zone! I love you!

And here is your current potential with the resources, experiences and current understanding you have at the moment:

 *Hello potential! I am excited about this possibility, are you?*

Now here is what they look like together:

 *Doesn't your comfort zone look nice and cosy... and small?!*

Now let us take a look at what happens when you step outside your comfort zone. Say you try a few new things, visited some new places, had some new experiences, spoke to different people, read something interesting, listened to something new, tried something that made you nervous, looked for tasks that raised your heartbeat slightly... this all sounds so exciting to me... but what about you?

If you were to take small steps outside your comfort zone you may notice that it would start to look like:

How does that diagram make you feel now? Still comfortable but perhaps now you experience feelings of achievement, success, happiness and joy. You feel like you have more 'space'. Like you take up more space! Yes, we want to take up more space. We want to be seen, heard and loved!

Let's look at when you keep stepping outside your comfort zone.

Now how does this diagram make you feel? Isn't it interesting how you start to think that there is not enough space. Or perhaps you feel like you are taking up too much space! You might hear your inner mean voice telling you to stay where you are, there is no need to get any bigger, if you do...you will reach your full potential.

Is this true?

Can you ever reach your full potential?

What would happen if the two circles were identical in size and matched each other perfectly? If I was to ask, what if you reached your full potential and felt like you had everything you ever wanted in life? What would you honestly say?

Yep, me too. I would want more. And that is okay. You can want more. I can want more. We can all have more. Because our potential is limitless. Our impact is limitless. Our opportunities are endless.

So, what happens when the two circles meet? Your next level. Your new comfort zone and new possibility for you highest potential.

Now look at the original diagram but with this perspective.

Do you look at this diagram with excitement rather than fear? Do you see the potential now, knowing that you have already 'passed a level' before? You have been passing levels all your life... ever since you started achieving those milestones when you were a baby! Somewhere along your timeline you have created the belief that stepping outside your comfort zone is not worth it. Accessing your highest potential is worth it and it plays a key role in creating the life you want to live!

Everything you have in your life right now is a product of what you have created. Your choices, your decisions, your thoughts and your actions. This is probably the hardest concept my coaching clients have to swallow when I work with them. Life can be pretty cruel sometimes and we may not have the luck we want at certain times. However, it all, unfortunately or fortunately, comes down to what you want to attract to your life. Have you ever thought about moving house and then started to see 'For Sale' signs everywhere you drive? Or perhaps you have been pregnant or were trying to fall pregnant and then all of a sudden you see women who are pregnant everywhere. At workshops I used to say that even when you started to think about the things you wanted or holidays you wanted to go on, you could start to see deals or advertisements on the TV or your phone. There are algorithms in your phone that can pick up on words you have typed or said out aloud whilst your phone or app is on and these algorithms can then line up the relevant advertisements, so use this to your advantage for the life you want to create!

You can access this level of magic in creating the life you want to live! If you imagine the person you want to be, the things you want to do and the things you want to have and the start embodying all those things right now, you will attract the same things into your life or at least take steps outside of your comfort zone to transport you to a level where they can be accessed.

This is a great time to revisit the Align section of this book to identify again what you really want in life and how you can incrementally make changes using your natural feminine energy cycle.

Chapter 27

How to Work Out What Your Shine Is

Take some time to think about what makes you happy. In order to shine brightly you need to feel like you are shining on the inside. When I ask my workshop participants how they want to feel, happy, is always one of the top three answers! So, if you want to shine from within, you need to do what makes you happy and that happiness will naturally project outwards.

When I was in high school, a group of my friends organised a Secret Santa. I remembered feeling so good about being asked if I wanted to join in with their Secret Santa (probably in my Spring Week) and then feeling like I should have said no when I had to organise the gift (probably in my Autumn Week) to then being highly emotional when I received my gift (yep, probably in my Winter Week). I received this yellow bear with 'happiness angel' written on the belly. I also remember asking the friend who got it for me (because seriously when does Secret Santa stay secret?) and why she got it for me because I was significantly disappointed that I did not get a candle and some body cream like I got my Secret Santa recipient. She replied that she went shopping and saw this bear hanging up and immediately thought of me because I am alway happy (boy, was she wrong) and I make others happy when they are around me. I have later learnt, like 20 years later, that this is my energy, the energy that others can feel. So, I aim to shine brightly. I aim to shine brightly for myself, my family and my community.

If you were to take a moment to work out what makes you happy could you list 10 things?
Out of those 10 on your list, how many also make others shine? Which ones just make you shine?
How can you incorporate more of these things on your 'Happy List' right now? Can you allocate some of these to your seasonal weeks?

We have spoken about how you can change your internal world to improve your external world. How can you feel like you are shining on the inside? Perhaps you just need a reset where you focus on yourself again and really prioritise your own health and wellbeing. Select one thing and focus on that. Do it well and find the consistency you would like to have it become a habit in your life. Then move on to the next one. I like to create a flow chart of the things I can do to really focus on how I can make my shine brighter by starting with my internal world.

You are in charge of making your shine bright. No one else can do it for you. They can do things that make your shine spark, but it is not long-lasting, and you end up requiring more validation of your worthiness (your shine). It is also not your job to continue the shine for others. You can ignite it, light it and inspire it, but it is not your responsibility to look after it. Not even your own children. Your job is to ensure you are keeping your own light bright. Your own shine is your own ability. By looking after your own light, you will inspire others to do the same, you might even give them the permission to do it if they are not able to give the permission to themselves. You will be leading by example and inspiring others along the way!

Receive a compliment, accept it and hear it, but don't hold onto it thinking you need to hear it again. Allow it to fill your cup and love tank but then do some more things to reinforce that that is also how you feel about yourself. For too long we have determined our worth according to what others think of us. What you think of yourself is all that matters. So, give yourself reasons to think highly of yourself. Pay attention to yourself. Look after yourself. Treat yourself nicely.

A lot of it comes down to getting to know yourself again. Who you were, who you are and who you want to be. What does your shine look like in all these situations? What lights you up? What impact did you make, what impact are you making now and what impact do you want to make? What do you want to be remembered for? And one that gets me every time: what do you want your kids to remember about you?

This is where your shine lies. Inside of you. Inside of your dreams. Right now. And in your highest potential. So, it is time now to let that shine out!

Chapter 28

Some Last Thoughts

TAKING YOUR SHINE FURTHER

I strongly believe all women should run a business. I am not a fan of calling it a side hustle or hobby. If you run a business, it is a business. If you have a product or service that you exchange for money, it is a business. There have been numerous times where I have felt like my business was not worthy because I also worked as a teacher. There is no set criteria on how much time you have to spend or how much money you need to make in order to called it a business. The aim for women to have a business is to create financial independence. There have been so many times I wished I had found my shine at a younger age and way before I had kids. That way I could have spent that time in my life (that season) building it to a point where it financially supported me so then when I did have children, I could choose to stay at home or go back to work with no consideration about money. It also takes a lot of time to create a community to share your shine in.

Please do not think that you have to turn your shine into

a money-making activity. That is not what I am saying at all. If there is one shine in particular that makes you happy and can make money—can you turn that into a business? Notice how I did not say profitable business. There is no need to place any expectation onto what your business will become, and I will explain this in more detail in my next book *She Energy for Women in Business*. For now, let's look at starting your business out of pure joy and excitement. Use this experience as its own personal development journey and another way to step outside your comfort zone. Look into personal branding as a business model rather than leading from the product or service. Who are you as a person? What do you have to offer? How can you help others? How do you serve? This is taking your shine one step further.

I would also like to encourage young women to embark on a journey of owning their own business from a very young age. There is something about the skills you acquire when you run your own business and not to mention when you earn your own money. Embedding this foundation at a young age can collectively release the freedom of all women all over the world. Imagine more conscious women with money who can make a bigger impact in the world! I also feel that this is necessary if women are in a position where they want to and can have babies. I did not realise the full effect that raising a family would have on my career and work. If I could go back, I would have started a business before having children, something that allowed me to have not only flexible hours but earn income as well. Women are often the ones who need to rework their schedules and aspirations when they become mothers, the ones who take the sick days when the children are unwell. This is a very general perspective, but I still think with valid reason. What if we could be financially independent and stepping outside our comfort zone whilst raising a family? To me, this is the clear definition of having it all! Having all that we want. Not relying on anyone else giving it to us and creating it for ourselves.

HOW SHE ENERGY CAN CHANGE THE WORLD

I am talking about collective energy here. If every woman in the world chose to utilise their natural feminine energy cycle and tapped into their *She Energy*, the collective power would be unstoppable. But even for me, I start to freak out about making a huge impact or difference because that means I have a lot of responsibility. But that is where I know that I am being led by my ego and not my heart. True change and impact starts within ourselves and then ripples out to those who are close to us. It is then the collective energy of our closest that makes a bigger change in our communities which then ripples out to other communities. We must start within before it flows externally.

If you were to list how you feel on a daily basis at present, how many emotions would be positive or negative? I could almost predict that 9 out of 10 women would have 'tired' written on their list. This is because today's society does not honour resting, and it certainly does not accommodate for the hormonal changes happening on a regular basis in our bodies. The 9 to 5 workday, the calendar months and even time in general were long ago created by society. What if we were to rewrite how we saw these measures of time? If we could change the way we work to accommodate our energy? Most of all, what if we were celebrated for having emotions and showing vulnerability rather than seeing it as a sign that we are approaching 'the time of the month'?

When women move forward, we should encourage those behind us to follow and seek the easier path, just because it was hard work for us does not mean that everyone else has to experience the hard road. If you allow someone else to follow you and then help them to move forward, you are collectively raising all women up. When all women seek and FEEL their potential, massive shifts and changes will occur.

Welcome to the Lead and Inspire Community! I am so thrilled to have you here! I am grateful for being part of your journey. My hope is that you feel unstoppable after reading this. That you feel unapologetically you! That you stop waiting for the time and create the opportunities. That you stop feeling like you don't have the energy and utilise your own natural energy cycle that is on repeat inside of you. That you now see that your highest potential is available and that stepping outside your comfort zone is really worth it. That you give yourself permission to stop and look after yourself. That you see you are worth your own time. And most of all, that you now see that your menstrual cycle is actually a superpower!

Thank you for being here!

What you can do right now with this knowledge?
Share it with your girlfriends.
Share it with your family.
Share it with your partner.
Share it with your team.
Share it in your business.
Share it with your colleagues.
Share it with your daughter.

Acknowledgements

I write this as I sit in my office, looking at my vision board and listening to my number one cheerleader husband, Ben. Our gorgeous children Ava and Rob get dinner and school lunches sorted. As I reflect on the items I have on my vision board, I realise, that although there are things on there that I am yet to achieve and places I still have to visit. Life is very sweet.

From a very young age I have been supported and encouraged to achieve my personal best. My wonderful parents, Gino and Anne, are the reason why I knew that I could reach for the stars and go for what I wanted because if I ever did fall, and I did, they would be there to catch me.

Thank you, Mum and Dad from the bottom of my heart. Thank you for my love of life, holidays, good food and family.

To my siblings, Benjamin, Mathew and Melissa, I know my teenage years were not my finest hour, but you really are amazing human beings. I am so very proud of you and love you all very much.

To Ben, babe, thank you for understanding that my crazy ideas and desire for more is all because I have so much to give.

Thank you for understanding that I know that we have an amazing life, and we are so very lucky and blessed but that I do need to be more, do more and have more. I am so very proud of all you have achieved, and I am so grateful for our relationship and life we have built and continue to build together. Thank you for making this dream come true! Love you always and forever.

Ava and Rob, my gorgeous children, I am so lucky to be your mum. Thank you for teaching me so much. I love our Team Terlick and I am so excited to enjoy the present moment with both of you.

I have been blessed with so many influential people in my life and along my life's journey so far. To my numerous Primary and High School teachers and sports coaches, thank you for supporting me as I navigated such an influential time, I truly feel like it was the foundations to who I am today. To Aleks Mutavdzic, Samantha Mudgway, Lorraine Lundie-Jenkins, Amy Jacobson, Ellie Swift, Andrea Gill, Jo Monkhouse, Rebecca Shelfhout, Suse Piek, Victoria Keep Tammy Tickel, you are all key people in my life, and all made an impact in your own special ways.

To my life-long friends; Billie Burvill, Tracey Bailey, Georgia Eddy, Sarah Goodliffe, Kimberley Bartlett you have been and continue to be there through each stage of my life.

To my Lead and Inspire Team, Gemma Wilson, Tracy Fryer, Aaron Divitini and my accountants at the McKinley Plowman Team, thank you for having such awesome zone of geniuses.

To the Lead and Inspire Community, I thank you! I thank you for getting involved and wanting more for yourself and your family. I love how you want more in life.

Thank you to my key founding members; Rachel Walker, Michelle Deering, Nadia Golding, Kristie Williams, Leanne Summers, Rachel Cusack-Kemp, Alexandra Baker, Sandrine Skane, Kelly Duggan, Wendy Godding, Tahlia Collins- you were the reason I knew I could keep going.

Natasha and her team at the kind press, my heart explodes for you all. I am so grateful for all your love and support with making this project come to life. Thank you to all that made this special project come to life. It has been so amazing to work with a company that is heart centred and cares about their clients.

And to you, yes you, I may know you and I may not just yet, but I am truly grateful for you. You are the reason I wrote this book. May you create the self-awareness that lights you up from the inside and shine brightly everywhere you go.

About the Author

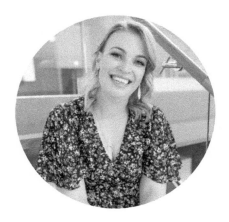

Jessica Terlick is an energetic presenter and empowerment coach who has been working in education for over a decade. She supports women and children in their personal development journeys through workshops, speaking events, online programs and coaching.

Spreading positive affirmations, Jessica provides women the space to recognise and harness their unique superpowers by prioritising self-care through time management, organisation skills, intention and reflection.

SheEnergy™ is for women who know they deserve more in life! Using the tools Jessica has outlined in *She Energy*, women can learn to utilise their natural feminine cycle to cultivate more time and energy.

Resources

Join our community, receive free materials!
You are invited to follow @jessicaterlick and join our *She Energy* community via www.jessicaterlick.com.au where you can also access free materials, including journals, affirmation cards and vision board cards — and more tools to support you along the way.

She Energy Membership
Explore *She Energy* further alongside this book, access the *She Energy* membership at www.jessicaterlick.com.au/membership

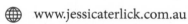 www.jessicaterlick.com.au
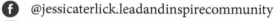 @jessicaterlick.leadandinspirecommunity
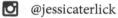 @jessicaterlick

She Energy
Tracking Journal

Is available to purchase alongside this book
as a tool to help you track your personal cycle,
including energy levels, eating patterns
and general mood.

The *She Energy Tracking Journal* invites you to better
understand how you work, so you can utilise your
time and energy.

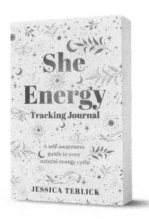

Lightning Source UK Ltd.
Milton Keynes UK
UKHW011830251122
412837UK00001B/167